KNOW THE FACTS

THE FACTS ABOUT
Mental Illness

Sara Rowe Mount

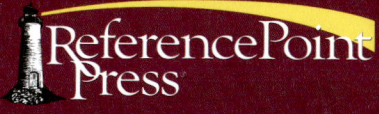

San Diego, CA

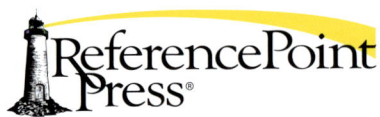

About the Author

Sara Rowe Mount writes articles and books for children and teens. Her passion for mental health advocacy stems from her own struggles with anxiety, obsessive-compulsive disorder, and depression. She lives in the Northeast with her husband, their daughter, and lots of books.

© 2026 ReferencePoint Press, Inc.
Printed in the United States

For more information, contact:
ReferencePoint Press, Inc.
PO Box 27779
San Diego, CA 92198
www.ReferencePointPress.com

ALL RIGHTS RESERVED.
No part of this work covered by the copyright hereon may be reproduced or used in any form or by any means—graphic, electronic, or mechanical, including photocopying, recording, taping, web distribution, or information storage retrieval systems—without the written permission of the publisher.

Picture Credits:
Cover: Chris Harwood/Shutterstock
 6: Pormezz/Shutterstock
10: Candy/Retriever/Shutterstock
12: BearPhotos/Shutterstock
19: DimaBerlin/Shutterstock
24: ThailandPrathankarnpap/Shutterstock
27: GailiLaud/Shutterstock
32: Rawpixel.com/Shutterstock
36: Create jobs 51/Shutterstock
40: Ron Adar/Shutterstock
44: Energeticgrandpa/Shutterstock
48: Monkey Business Images/Shutterstock
50: 1st Footage/Shutterstock
54: Vincent Dimilio/Shutterstock

LIBRARY OF CONGRESS CATALOGING-IN-PUBLICATION DATA

Names: Mount, Sara Rowe, author.
Title: The facts about mental illness / by Sara Rowe Mount.
Description: San Diego, CA : ReferencePoint Press, Inc., 2025. | Series: Know the facts | Includes bibliographical references and index. | Audience term: Teenagers
Identifiers: LCCN 2024053809 (print) | LCCN 2024053810 (ebook) | ISBN 9781678210427 (library binding) | ISBN 9781678210434 (ebook)
Subjects: LCSH: Mental illness--Juvenile literature.
Classification: LCC RC460.2 .M68 2025 (print) | LCC RC460.2 (ebook) | DDC 616.89--dc23/eng/20241218
LC record available at https://lccn.loc.gov/2024053809
LC ebook record available at https://lccn.loc.gov/2024053810

CONTENTS

Introduction   4
Mental Illness Beyond the Numbers

Chapter One   8
Misunderstanding Mental Illness

Chapter Two   21
The Challenges of Getting Care

Chapter Three   34
Mental Illness and Violence

Chapter Four   46
Mental Illness and Homelessness

Source Notes   57
For Further Research   60
Index   62

INTRODUCTION

Mental Illness Beyond the Numbers

James Reed's life began to fall apart in his late forties. For thirty years he had managed a series of gas stations, until the job became too much for him. Then he lost a subsequent job for repeatedly not showing up to work. What was keeping him from work and from his life was mental illness. "I was completely depressed all the time, barely functioning, barely getting to work, barely getting to family get-togethers," he reflects on that time. "I didn't want to be awake. I was taking a lot of sleeping pills."[1] After a period of unemployment, his family kicked him out of their house, and he found himself with nowhere to live. He began sleeping in front of a local library, a quiet place that felt safer than other locations.

While on the street, Reed had his first encounter with mental health treatment. A mobile medical unit at a shelter asked about his mental health. The staff gave him a tablet and connected him with a therapist who could conduct online sessions. "Then I could do it anywhere I wanted to," Reed says. "I just had to show up on time every two weeks. Video—wow. That helped a lot."[2] Now Reed lives with one of his sisters, with whom he was able to reconnect over email.

Accessing Treatment

For Sarah Erdreich, a visit to the emergency room (ER) led her to be admitted to a psychiatric hospital. After being diagnosed with breast cancer and undergoing radiation, a mastectomy, and reconstructive surgery, the painful recovery had taken a toll both physically and mentally. She was anxious and depressed, some days barely able to leave her bed. She had been trying to find a psychiatrist, but many doctors were not taking new patients. Often, she was just added to another long waiting list. Erdreich began to feel desperate. The psychiatric hospital was able to prescribe her an antidepressant and get her an appointment with an outpatient psychiatrist. Knowing that she was finally going to get help was as much of a relief as the antidepressant, but the entire experience felt bizarre. "I'd always assumed that being admitted to a psychiatric ward was something that only happened when you were suicidal or had a mental breakdown," Erdreich says. "I wasn't ashamed of being in a psych ward, but I couldn't ignore the fact that I'd had to step out of my life in order to get help. . . . I'd had to deliberately leave my family and home to get treatment as quickly as possible."[3]

Difficulty accessing treatment is a common problem for those with mental illness. The expense of mental health care is another barrier that those with mental illness often encounter. Avery, who lives in Texas and believes that their location also impacts the quality and high cost of health care, has had to go without mental health care on numerous occasions. In their area, therapy is over $100 a session, and the prescription medication for their bipolar disorder costs $200. "Unfortunately, due to financial constraints, there are times when I cannot afford to purchase [medication] for several months," Avery says. "This situation leaves me in a state of turmoil and emotional distress, all because I cannot consistently afford the medication throughout the year."[4] While Avery believes that therapy could be extremely beneficial, it is simply unobtainable when they cannot even afford medication some months.

> "I'd always assumed that being admitted to a psychiatric ward was something that only happened when you were suicidal or had a mental breakdown."[3]
>
> —Sarah Erdreich, an individual with mental illness

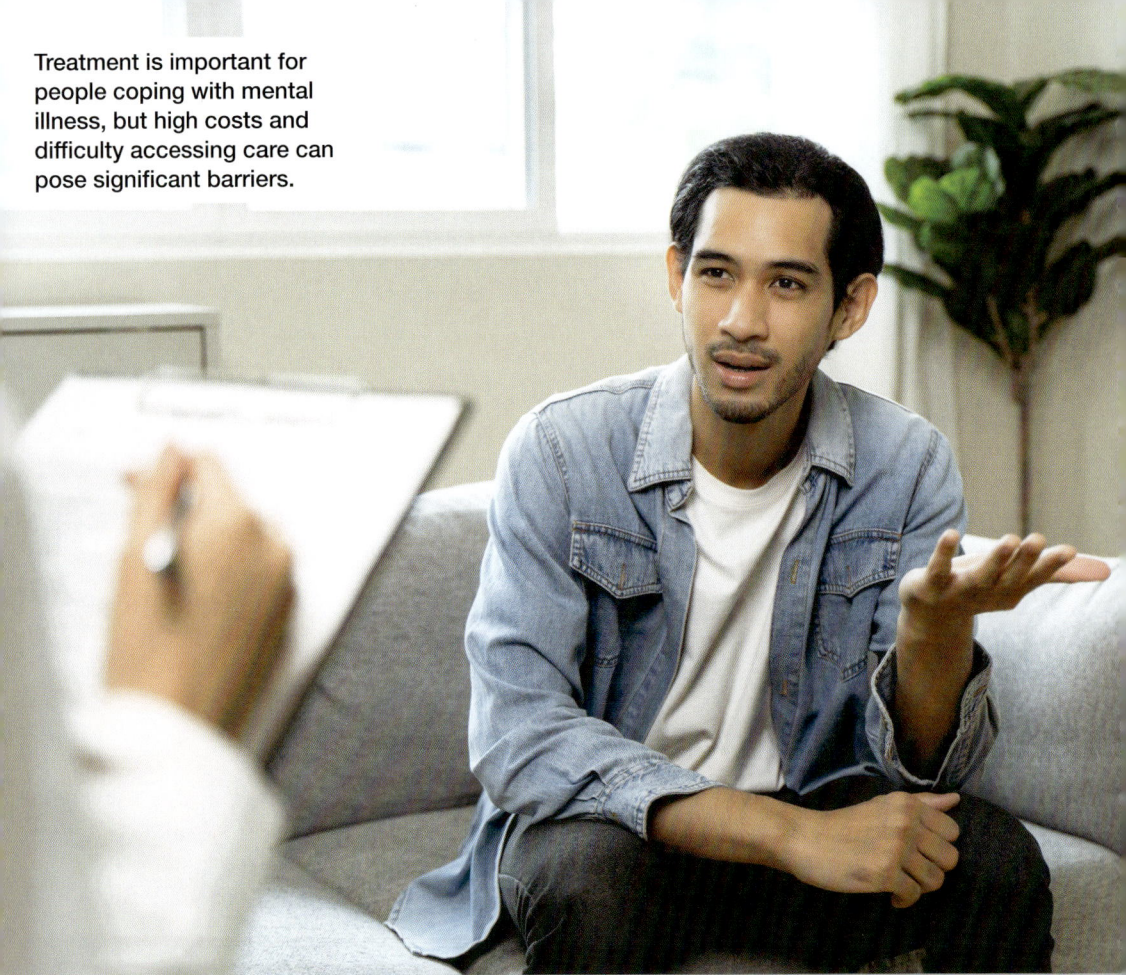

Treatment is important for people coping with mental illness, but high costs and difficulty accessing care can pose significant barriers.

The Problem with Stereotypes

Encounters with those who are mentally ill, messaging from social media or peers, and media coverage can all lead to internalizing stereotypes and stigmas associated with mental illness. A homeless person muttering while passing on the street might color a person's perception of both the homeless and the mentally ill. Movies may form the only understanding of how psychiatric hospitals operate and who ends up in them. An authority figure's statement on the news about where the blame lies for a school shooting can strengthen the public's belief in the connection between violence and mental illness.

Even language can impact how Americans feel about mental illness and those who have been diagnosed. Describing people and their behavior as crazy, unhinged, deranged, or psycho continues to feed stereotypes about how those with mental illness behave. Ultimately, these stereotypes have a very real impact on the lives of people living with mental illness. Connecting mental illness with insanity can result in individuals being reluctant to seek out treatment for fear of being labeled crazy. Individuals with mental illness also can be subject to judgment and discrimination even in their doctor's office. But false or inaccurate stereotypes also have an impact on health care policies that are enacted and funded, which can make it difficult for those in need to access treatment.

The prevalence of stigma and stereotypes and the impact this can have on the individuals suffering from mental illness make knowing the facts about mental illness important. Dispelling false information about what it is like to live with mental illness is key to ensuring that all people are able to receive adequate and affordable mental health care and feel comfortable seeking it out.

CHAPTER ONE

Misunderstanding Mental Illness

When Putri Surya reflects on her childhood and teen years, she remembers them being dominated by anxiety and depression. When she finally had the courage around age thirteen to tell her parents that she was struggling, they were less than supportive because of their own beliefs about mental illness. "My parents are practicing Muslims who believed my mental illness was just all in my head and if I was closer to God, it would all just go away," Surya says. "I would read the Quran and pray as they suggested, but it just made me more angry at God because I felt like I wasn't making any progress."[5] While they did make appointments with psychiatrists and therapists for her, initially they did not want her to be prescribed medication for her anxiety and depression.

Eventually, Surya was able to find a therapist who was the right fit, and the therapist was able to convince her parents that medication was a key part of her treatment plan. "Even though my parents, especially my dad still thinks having a strong faith is the best solution to mental illness, their open mind literally saved my life," Surya says. "Anxiety and depression is still something I have to battle everyday, but the patience and understanding of everyone around me has made it a lot easier."[6]

Misinformation about what mental illness is and how it should be treated is rampant, especially on social media. For teenagers, many of whom spend hours a day on the internet and browsing and posting on social media, this can be especially impactful.

Stereotypes and stigma about mental illness that are developed from misinformation can make it difficult for those experiencing symptoms to seek out and access care. They can also lead to quick judgments about those suffering from mental illness and how they do or should behave. These stereotypes and judgments have far-reaching consequences, impacting laws, policies, and the care available for those suffering.

What Is Mental Illness?

Mental illnesses, according to the American Psychiatric Association, "are health conditions involving changes in emotion, thinking or behavior (or a combination of these)."[7] They can affect an individual's quality of life, impacting the ability to work, go to school, care for children, and maintain healthy relationships. While mental health is often viewed as separate from physical health, they are very interconnected. Struggling with one's physical health can often result in mental health conditions, and mental illnesses often have physical symptoms as well as emotional and cognitive ones.

The 2023 National Survey on Drug Use and Health found that 22.8 percent of American adults suffered from mental illness and 5.7 percent from serious mental illness, which was defined as "[having] any mental, behavioral, or emotional disorder that substantially interfered with or limited one or more major life activities."[8] Among younger Americans, 23.4 percent of adolescents aged twelve to seventeen were found to suffer from a substance abuse disorder, mental illness, or both. Those who used and abused substances were more than twice as likely to have experienced a depressive episode than those who had not.

Mental health professionals are authorities in diagnosing mental illness. These professionals include psychologists, licensed therapists, and psychiatrists—medical doctors who can both provide psychotherapy and prescribe medication. To make a

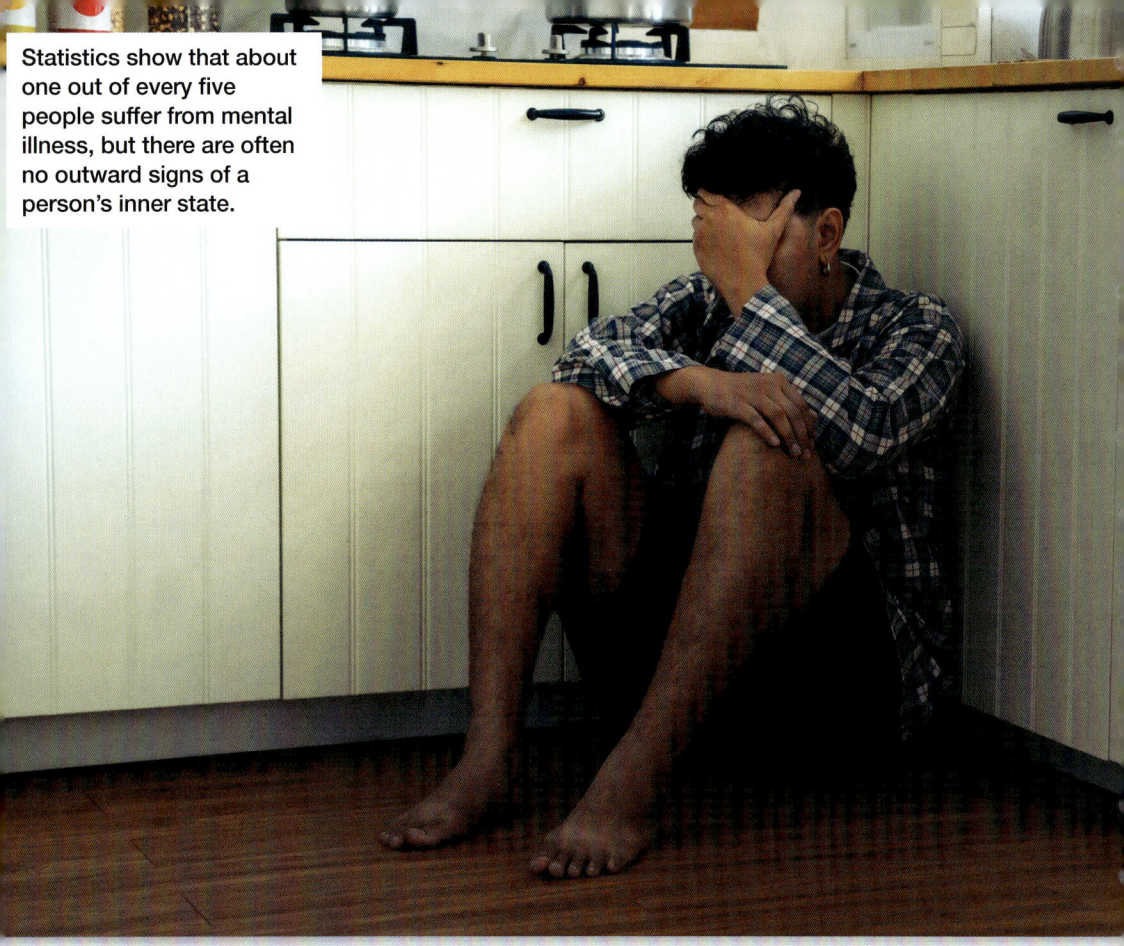

Statistics show that about one out of every five people suffer from mental illness, but there are often no outward signs of a person's inner state.

diagnosis, mental health professionals will gather their patients' medical history, symptoms, and family history and responses to psychological questionnaires. They typically consult with the patients to hear their stories and question them about their experiences and concerns. "Skilled diagnosticians not only consider the answers to all such questions in establishing a diagnosis, they also take into account a person's emotional tone, demeanor, attitude, appearance, and responsiveness," says Hara Estroff Marano, an editor for *Psychology Today*. "What's more, they are also assessing a person's mental status, such as the ability to think clearly, remember facts, and sustain attention."[9]

While there are currently no medical tests that can diagnose mental illness, blood work or other tests can be used to rule out specific physiological causes or to determine whether another medical condition could be exacerbating mental health symptoms. The fifth edition of the *Diagnostic and Statistical Manual of Mental Disorders* (DSM-5), developed by the American Psychiatric Association, contains diagnostic criteria that helps mental health professionals determine diagnoses for each individual.

The most common mental illnesses in the United States are major depressive disorder and anxiety disorders. The 2023 National Survey on Drug Use and Health found that 5.9 percent of adults and 18.1 percent of adolescents experienced a major depressive episode. Those with depression encounter periods of low mood, loss of interest or enjoyment in life and preferred activities, and low self-esteem. They also suffer physical symptoms such as disturbances to sleeping and eating patterns, aches and pains,

Religious Beliefs as a Barrier to Treatment

While most people no longer believe that mental illness is a result of demonic possession, religious beliefs can still have a great impact on what many people believe about the root causes of mental illness and treatment. Many religions, especially more insular or fundamentalist sects, teach that mental illness is not an illness but the result of sinful behavior or a lack of faith. Those experiencing symptoms of anxiety or depression, for example, might be encouraged to pray more, consult their religion's holy books, or examine their life for behaviors that may be separating them from their god. Often, consulting medical professionals such as a psychiatrist or psychologist is either discouraged or forbidden in favor of receiving counseling from a priest or other clergy member. In a 2019 *Psychiatric Services* article, psychiatrist John R. Peteet stated:

> The Biblical Counseling . . . movement, which, in contending that truth can be known literally only through revelation in scripture, rejects mainstream psychology and psychiatry as humanistic, secular, and antithetical to Christianity. . . . For example, a woman with complex PTSD, nightmares, and hypersensitivity to suspected abuse was encouraged to think about her symptoms as demonic in origin and to tell negative thoughts to "go back to the pit of hell."

John R. Peteet, "Approaching Religiously Reinforced Mental Health Stigma: A Conceptual Framework," *Psychiatric Services*, June 12, 2019. https://psychiatryonline.org.

low energy, and difficulty concentrating. The Centers for Disease Control and Prevention's 2023 National Health Interview Survey found that 12.5 percent of adults were regularly experiencing feelings of anxiety. Individuals with anxiety disorders face ongoing, chronic worry and fear that is either generalized or specified, such as discomfort in social situations. Other symptoms may be similar to those experienced with depression but in addition include racing thoughts, fatigue, digestive issues, and feelings of restlessness and irritability. Other mental disorders classified in the DSM-5 include eating disorders, substance abuse disorders, bipolar disorder, obsessive-compulsive disorder, and gender dysphoria.

Among the most severe mental illnesses are schizophrenia and other psychotic disorders, which studies have estimated affect somewhere between 0.25 and 0.64 percent of the population in the United States. The symptoms for schizophrenia include hallucinations, or seeing or hearing things that are not actually there, and delusions, false beliefs that impair trust and interper-

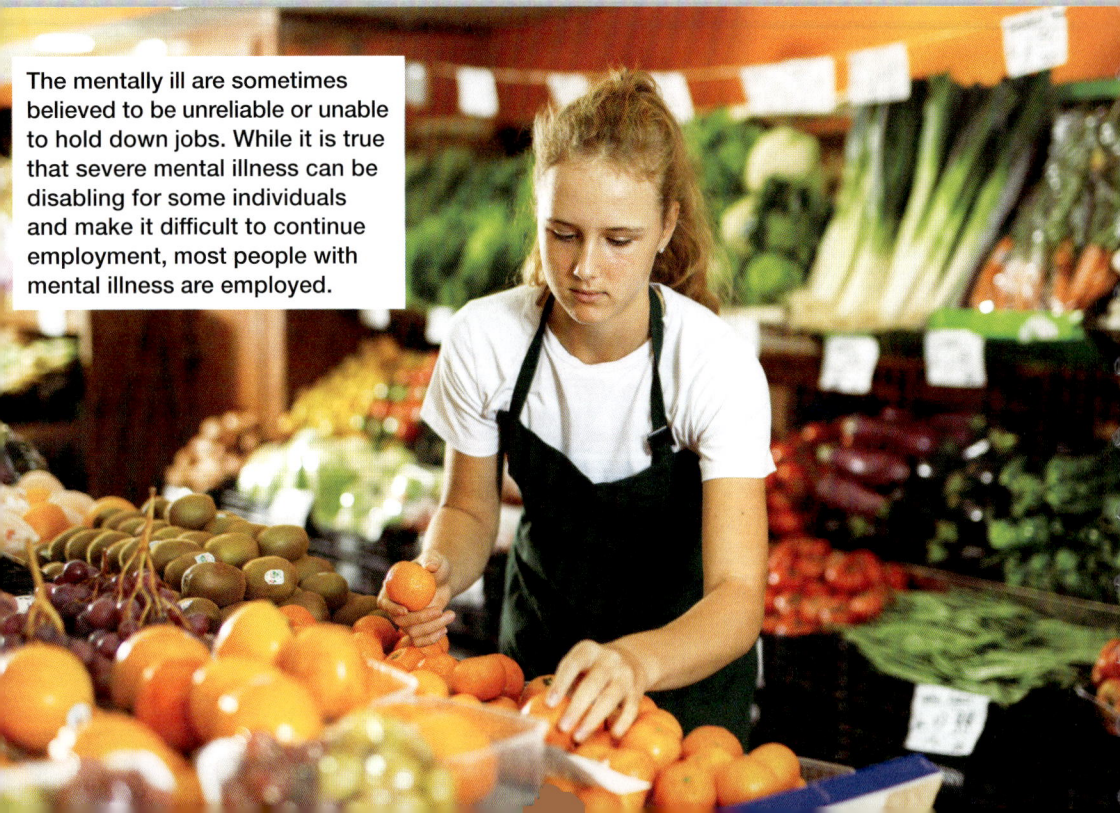

The mentally ill are sometimes believed to be unreliable or unable to hold down jobs. While it is true that severe mental illness can be disabling for some individuals and make it difficult to continue employment, most people with mental illness are employed.

sonal relationships and make successfully navigating everyday life challenging. Because of these atypical behaviors and cognitive processes, people who suffer from schizophrenia or other psychotic disorders are likely to be dismissed as violent, dangerous, untreatable, and worthy of institutionalization. However, many individuals who suffer from psychotic disorders receive professional help and work to manage their symptoms.

Challenging Stereotypes About Mental Illness

Even as health professionals and others seek to destigmatize mental illnesses, those who struggle with them have been subject to stereotyping and societal ignorance for thousands of years. From the earliest civilizations through the seventeenth century, mental illnesses were commonly considered the result of possession by evil spirits or punishment by divine beings. Treatment for the mentally ill in the Western world was often provided by religious communities, including monasteries, and exorcisms were practiced, among other now debunked treatments. Asylums and mental institutions often isolated and housed away from public view those with mental illnesses, along with vagrants, the physically disabled, and others who did not adapt to societal norms.

Over time, reforms turned the care for the mentally ill over to those with medical expertise, and that changed how some caregivers viewed the causes of mental illness—even if it did not necessarily change the treatment regimen. As Andrew Scull, author of *Madness in Civilization*, says, "By the time we reached the 18th century, most people have adopted a medical perspective on madness and see it rooted in the same general kinds of pathology as illness. . . . It's a mix because medicine is holistic at that time, and it incorporates both the realm of the psychological and the physical."[10] However, the medical community still persisted in both abusive and torturous treatments that often left patients traumatized.

Although knowledge about the human brain and mental illness have grown in the intervening centuries, many disparaging stereotypes persist. For instance, mental illness is still considered distinct from physical illness and often viewed as less severe or worthy of attention because it is not generally life-threatening. Many people also believe that recovery from mental illness is within the control of the individual diagnosed with it. Some maintain that mental illness is a result of moral weakness or character flaws rather than a complex combination of genes, adverse experiences, upbringing, and other factors. The website Medical News Today corrects this view, insisting, "Mental health disorders are illnesses, not signs of poor character. Similarly, people with, for instance, depression, cannot 'snap out of it' any more than someone with diabetes or psoriasis can immediately recover from their condition."[11] Those who preach that mental struggles can be resolved by willpower often deter individuals from seeking help and getting treatment.

> "Mental health disorders are illnesses, not signs of poor character. Similarly, people with, for instance, depression, cannot 'snap out of it' any more than someone with diabetes or psoriasis can immediately recover from their condition."[11]
>
> —Medical News Today

Similarly, those who are mentally ill are often believed to be unreliable, erratic, and unable to hold down jobs. The facts, however, do not support this perspective. While it is true that severe mental illness can be disabling for some individuals and make it difficult to continue employment, most people with mental illness are employed. A 2014 study by Alison Luciano and Ellen Meara of the 2009 and 2010 National Survey on Drug Use and Health found that the employment rate was 75.9 percent for those reporting no mental illness, 68.8 percent for those with mild mental illness, 62.7 percent for those with moderate mental illness, and 54.5 percent for those with serious mental illness.

Portrayals of the Mentally Ill as Violent

Beyond accusations of unemployability and moral failings, news coverage of mental illness has contributed to the belief that the mentally ill are dangerous and violent. News stories involving violent crimes—especially gun crimes—often highlight the investigation into the perpetrator's mental health. While some mental illnesses can impair judgment, the amplification of a connection between mental health issues and violence reinforces the message that people with mental illness are dangerous and prone to aggression.

The American Psychological Association has been studying why such misinformation is so easy to absorb as factual. Its researchers contend that the brain focuses only on understanding new information, not determining whether it can be trusted or is accurate. Questioning the validity of information comes later, through critical thinking. The researchers also point out that many factors influence how information is accepted and processed, explaining, "People are more likely to believe false statements that appeal to emotions such as fear and outrage. They are also more likely to believe . . . repeated information, even when it contradicts their prior knowledge."[12]

The Impact of Social Media

Many of the falsehoods related to mental illness are spread via social media. These platforms provide a stage for every kind of voice, from vetted, legacy news sources, to individuals with opinions, to artificial bots designed to spread misinformation. And social media has replaced television, radio, and print news as the primary means by which people receive information. A 2024 Pew Research Center study found that 52 percent of TikTok users were getting news on the platform (a 30 percent increase since 2020), only topped by 59 percent of Twitter users.

Social media, however, is rampant with misinformation that can be easily spread to millions of users. While many platforms use artificial intelligence to flag false or misleading statements, it is challenging to stamp out all misinformation or remove it fast enough to prevent some users from seeing it and passing it on, especially to others who already echo their views. The American Psychological Association asserts, "Social media typically lacks the oversight and safeguards of legacy media to prevent and correct false claims. Its algorithms and peer-to-peer sharing model are a perfect setup for misinformation to be shared widely, especially within the echo chambers that form online."[13]

On social media, individuals can share anything and present it as fact. The result is often that this information is spread quickly. Jeremy Tyler, an assistant professor of clinical psychiatry, says, "As we know on social media, with enough people saying it, then people may accept false information as fact."[14] Most of the information about mental illness available on social media platforms is not being shared by licensed mental health professionals, which increases the likelihood that it may be false or misleading. An analysis of 168 TikTok videos about cognitive behavioral therapy published in the *Journal of Medical Internet Research* in 2023 found that 37.5 percent were posted by nonprofessionals (such as former patients) and 19.1 percent by mental health coaches, who are not licensed mental health professionals. Of these 168 videos, 22.6 percent provided mixed or negative feedback on cognitive behavioral therapy, and they were the ones with the highest engagement in the form of comments.

Even if information is not blatantly false, social media posts can often contain only one individual's personal experience of mental illness. While sharing these personal experiences can be empowering and inspiring, they are limited to that singular perspective. In addition, people detailing their own symptoms and treatments has also resulted in higher rates of self-diagnosis, especially among children and teenagers. After viewing content about another teen's diagnosis, symptoms, or choice of treat-

A Teen's Perspective on Mental Illness Stigma

"Pop culture portrayals of mental illness frequently highlight the extremes. . . . Distorted societal perception of mental health issues can diminish the lived reality of people. When disorders are portrayed as manageable, seeking support within social circles can seem extreme. However, when disorders are shown as dangerous, treatment can feel premature or unnecessary. These narratives reinforce the notion that therapy is for those in immediate crisis, not also for those seeking support in managing their ongoing mental wellbeing. In this sense, therapy has become stigmatized. Acknowledging that you go to therapy risks implying an acute event, a point teenagers seeking help may not feel they have reached. . . . The conversation about mental health issues needs to shift. Normalizing is not the same as destigmatizing. Mental health issues should be accepted, but their impact should not be diminished. Four years ago, I should not have feared going to therapy for my mental health issues. I needed someone to sit me down and tell me that, although it seemed scary, it was okay, and there were people ready to support me. We can change the dialogue around mental health stigma, normalizing getting help, not normalizing silent struggling."

—Dresden, a teen with mental health issues

Dresden, "Normalize the Care to Destigmatize the Conditions," National Institute on Minority Health and Health Disparities, May 31, 2024. www.nimhd.nih.gov.

ment, young viewers might determine that they identify with that experience, even if they have not been through a proper diagnosis. Mental health providers worry that when there is an overreliance on social media content, fewer sufferers will seek professional diagnosis and treatment. Jennifer Katzenstein of Johns Hopkins All Children's Hospital has encountered this reliance on oversimplifications and blind trust in social media, especially among young patients' understanding of obsessive-compulsive disorder and bipolar disorder. She says:

> Adolescents are in a phase of identity formation, autonomy development, and self-discovery, seeking validation and understanding. The open discussions on social media

provide them with relatable content, fostering a sense of belonging and reducing the feeling of isolation. . . . Using social media platforms for self-diagnosis may lead to incorrect perceptions of one's mental health and as a result can cause unnecessary stress and anxiety. This can also delay access to appropriate interventions.[15]

While there is undoubtedly harm that can be caused by sharing and spreading misinformation about mental illness on social media, these platforms also have been used as tools to raise awareness and create community among those diagnosed with mental illnesses. When information is shared by reputable sources, such as licensed mental health professionals and mental health nonprofits, there are public benefits. Connecting with other individuals who may be experiencing similar feelings and symptoms from mental illness can reduce feelings of isolation. And concerned organizations can direct individuals to resources that will help them access treatment.

> "Using social media platforms for self-diagnosis may lead to incorrect perceptions of one's mental health and as a result can cause unnecessary stress and anxiety. This can also delay access to appropriate interventions."[15]
>
> —Jennifer Katzenstein, psychologist

Effects of Misinformation

Information about mental health and mental illness is more readily available in the digital age, but misinformation and oversimplification continue to feed stereotypes and engender feelings of shame. This may lead those with mental illnesses to try to manage symptoms on their own and potentially never seek treatment. It can also result in sufferers facing intense feelings of isolation and loneliness because they may feel hopeless and unable to connect with people around them if they fear judgment or being dismissed.

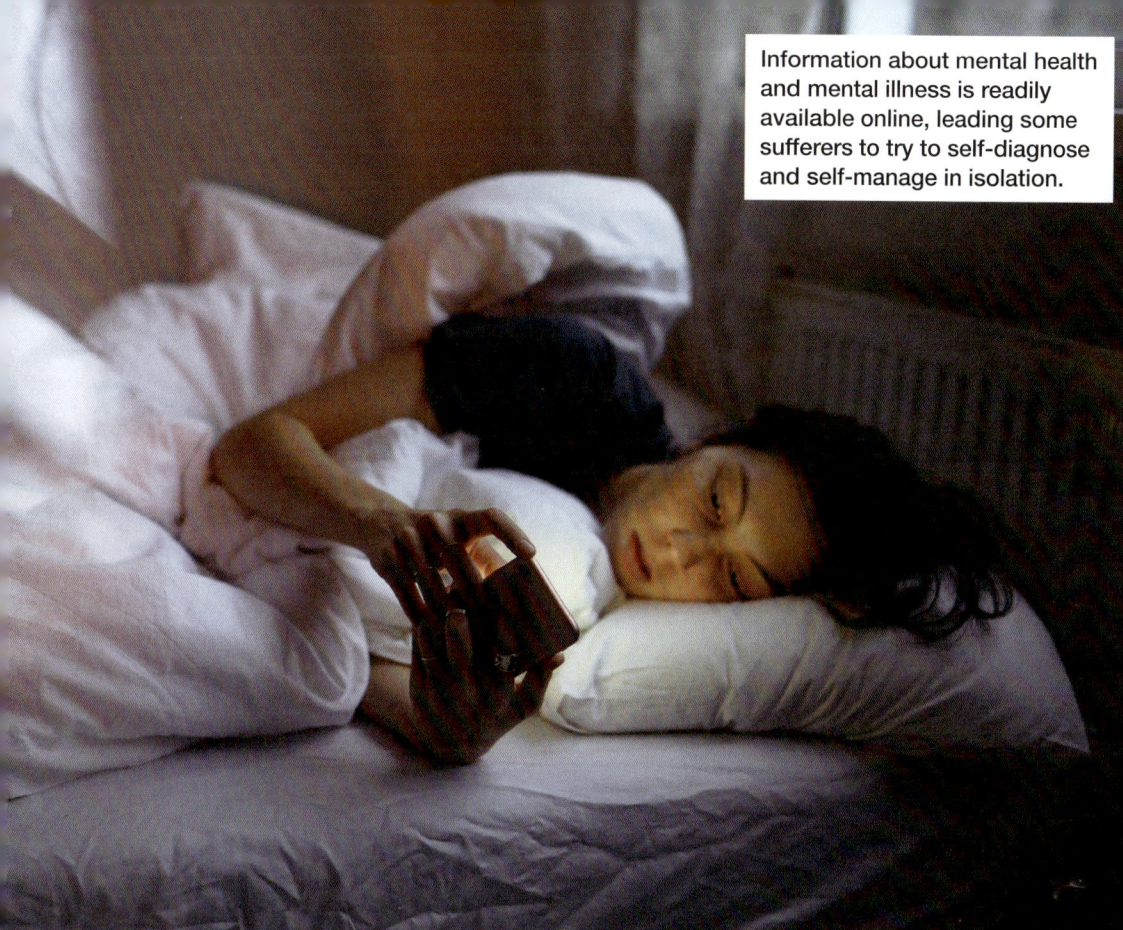

Information about mental health and mental illness is readily available online, leading some sufferers to try to self-diagnose and self-manage in isolation.

There is also the desire to hide symptoms or not disclose a diagnosis in settings like school, college, and the workplace. Fear of discrimination, of asking for accommodations, and of being passed over for jobs and promotions are common worries for those in educational and work environments. While the Americans with Disabilities Act of 1990 is supposed to protect American employees and students with mental illnesses from discrimination and harassment, it cannot prevent it. For example, in 2021 the US Equal Employment Opportunity Commission received eighty-four hundred charges from employees who believed they had been discriminated against because of their mental illness or substance abuse disorder.

Misinformation and the resulting stigma surrounding mental illness can even affect medical treatment that patients receive.

Doctors might make snap judgments about patients or dismiss their symptoms. Veronica Karp, who has personally experienced this discrimination in her own health care, says:

> [A 2000 study] found that doctors are less likely to believe that a patient's severe headaches or abdominal pain are symptoms of a serious illness and order further diagnostic evaluations if the patient has a history of depression. Despite their education and expertise, doctors aren't immune to implicit bias and actually perpetuate stigma against mental health at equal or higher rates compared to the general public.[16]

Subsequent studies have demonstrated that this remains the case not only in the medical community but also among health insurers and government policymakers.

Such institutional stigma can be a barrier to available and affordable treatment options. For example, health insurance companies continue to treat mental and physical illness coverage differently, prioritizing treatment for physical illnesses and disorders, while often making mental health treatment more expensive to the consumer and compensating licensed mental health providers less than other medical professionals for the care they provide.

A survey conducted by the Harris Poll on behalf of the American Psychological Association in 2018 found that while 87 percent of those surveyed believed that having a mental health disorder was nothing to be ashamed of, 39 percent admitted that they would view someone differently if they knew that person had a disorder. Thus, while there has been improvement in raising awareness about mental illness, misinformation and stigma still often control the rhetoric surrounding it.

CHAPTER TWO

The Challenges of Getting Care

Americans have begun to recognize the importance of prioritizing mental health and making sure all have access to treatment. An increasing understanding of how the human brain works and communicates with the body has led to more progressive beliefs about mental illness and how to treat it. Ineffective and often harmful treatments have been replaced with those that are based in scientific research and give individuals with mental illness the opportunity to live full lives. However, while treatment on a whole has improved, finding affordable, equitable mental health care is still challenging.

Accessing Medications

In America mental illness treatment occurs largely on an outpatient basis. Often, an individual first undertakes a screening with a primary care physician, such as a family medicine doctor, pediatrician, or OB-GYN. These doctors can assess symptoms, make a diagnosis, and prescribe medication if needed. For those experiencing mental illness, visiting a primary care physician can be a good alternative to trying to find a psychiatrist, since the number of psychiatrists has been on the decline since well before the COVID-19 pandemic highlighted the wide-ranging need for mental health care. Still, for individuals who are experiencing more severe symptoms or have tried several medications without effect, seeking out the expertise of a psychiatrist is worthwhile.

Both psychiatrists and primary care doctors can prescribe drug treatments to patients as part of outpatient care. Drugs developed to treat mental illnesses, such as antidepressants for depression and milder anxiety, antipsychotics for schizophrenia, and mood stabilizers for bipolar disorder attempt to address some of the biological causes of mental illness. However, unlike medications developed for physical ailments and diseases, prescribed drugs for mental illnesses still carry a stigma. This is in part because they are linked to psychiatric ailments and because researchers often argue that they are overprescribed and, in some cases, used as the sole treatment for an illness. Anne Harrington, a professor of the history of science at Harvard University, adds that students taking her course, Madness and Medicine, are wary because they are "growing up with messaging that tells them there's a lot to distrust when it comes to psychiatry and that Big Pharma is out to trick us all."[17]

Medication is not always the best choice for every individual struggling with mental illness, whether because of the mildness of their mental illness symptoms, the side effects the person has experienced, or poor interactions with other medication he or she is taking. For mental illnesses with more severe symptoms, medication is a key part of treatment to manage symptoms and improve the patient's quality of life. However, the combination of medication and psychotherapy is considered the most effective treatment plan for most individuals with mental illness. A 2020 analysis of 101 trials published in *World Psychiatry* found that patients with depression were 27 percent more likely to respond to this combination than to therapy alone and 25 percent more likely than those receiving only drug treatment. The analysis authors concluded, "These findings suggest that guidelines should recommend combined treatment as the first option in the treatment of depression and, because of the higher acceptability, may recommend psychotherapy before pharmacotherapy, depending on the preferences of patients."[18]

Inpatient and Outpatient Therapies

Medication in conjunction with therapy sessions form the basis of good outpatient mental health care. Cognitive behavioral therapy (CBT) is the most common therapy method, as well as the one that has been proved most effective for patients who suffer anxiety, depression, eating disorders, and other mental illnesses. CBT encourages patients to identify thought patterns that are false or distorted and how these are negatively affecting behavior. Those in CBT and other types of therapy work with the guidance of their therapist to break these harmful thought patterns and behaviors and to continue practicing these skills outside of therapy sessions. A patient experiencing anxiety might learn ways to identify patterns of overgeneralizing or responding to life with the fear that the worst may occur. And in the moment, a patient can focus on breathing and other relaxation techniques to respond to anxious feelings. Someone struggling with depression or an eating disorder may work on identifying negative thoughts, which can trigger harmful behaviors. Doing this can create space to focus on building self-esteem.

> "[Mental health] guidelines should recommend combined treatment as the first option in the treatment of depression and, because of the higher acceptability, may recommend psychotherapy before pharmacotherapy, depending on the preferences of patients."[18]
>
> —*World Psychiatry*

Mental health inpatient treatment and residential treatment facilities serve the needs of those struggling with substance abuse disorders, eating disorders, and other mental illnesses for which outpatient treatment has proved ineffective or for those who need immediate intervention. Patients may also be recommended for inpatient treatment if they are determined to be a safety risk to themselves or others. Residential programs range from three days to three months, depending on the issue and level of crisis. Some patients may be referred to a short-stay rehab center, while others might require a lengthier stay at a psychiatric hospital. Common

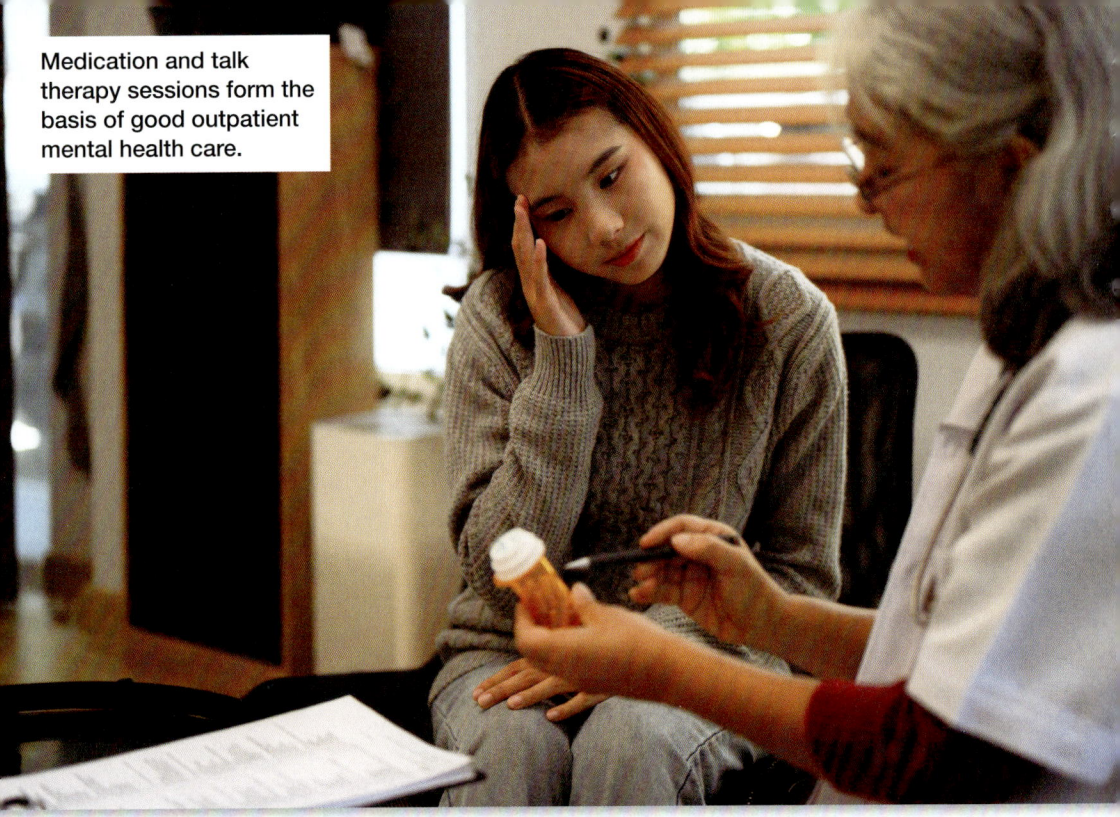

Medication and talk therapy sessions form the basis of good outpatient mental health care.

treatments in these residential programs include therapy sessions and activities to allay patients' mental distress and teach coping skills. Some facilities even offer day programs in which patients receive three to eight hours of therapy and other programming without an overnight stay.

Practitioner Shortages Prove a Barrier to Treatment

For those with mental illness, accessing both outpatient and inpatient treatment in the United States can be challenging. A national survey conducted by the actuary consulting firm Milliman in 2021 found that only 33 percent of those diagnosed with a mental health disorder received treatment from a behavioral health specialist in the year after receiving that diagnosis. This percentage was lower in certain states, such as Texas (22 percent) and Alabama (23.6 percent). One of the largest barriers to treatment is simply that there are shortages in the number of mental health professionals and facilities serving the number of Americans that need mental health care. The same Milliman report also discovered by combining Health Resources and Services Administration (HRSA) and US Census Bureau data that "174.7 million people (52.7% of the U.S. population) live in counties that are entirely designated as shortage areas, and only 23.7 million people (7.2%) live in counties that are not at all designated as shortage areas. The remaining 132.8 million people (40.1%) live in counties that are partly designated as shortage areas."[19] The HRSA has estimated that seventy-four hundred additional mental health care professionals are needed simply to meet the current national demand.

There are also more patients in need of care than ever. The Substance Abuse and Mental Health Services Administration found that there was an almost 30 percent increase in adults with diagnosed mental illness from 2008 to 2019, a rise of 39.8 million to 51.5 million. And with fewer psychologists, practitioners are often working longer hours and either cannot take on any additional

A Teen's Experience in the ER

"For seven days, I sat in an empty room with just my thoughts, in the moments I most needed support. At first, I was angry at the doctors. Every 'no,' every 'we don't know when,' every 'we'll let you know when we find out more' felt like a stone added to my already sinking ship. . . . Couldn't they do anything at all? . . . Unfortunately, my experience is not unique, and is in fact quite common. The mental health system is in disarray, and desperately needs to be changed. With waiting times years long to see a specialist proactively, the hospital system now acting on crisis is severely overloaded. There isn't enough funding, not enough doctors or therapists, especially not enough social workers, and not enough safe places for individuals, particularly teens, to go when they need it. This is a problem that is only getting worse. Change is going to take time, but we don't have that time. . . . The reason for that is simply the scope of the issue. It is not a problem with the people, it is a problem with the system."

—Maya, teen with mental illness

Maya, "Speaking Up for a Change," National Institute on Minority Health and Health Disparities, May 31, 2024. www.nimhd.nih.gov.

patients or maintain waiting lists in hopes of future openings. The 2022 COVID-19 Practitioner Impact Survey by the American Psychological Association discovered that 60 percent of psychologists could not take any more patients. Of the 38 percent that maintained waiting lists, 32 percent had ten to forty-nine people on their waiting list, and 10 percent had over fifty individuals hoping to get appointments. For those seeking treatment, not only will encountering provider after provider without any openings mean that they are not able to receive treatment, but the frustration, discouragement, and anger resulting from the process can often have a negative impact on their mental illness symptoms.

The time-intensive process of searching for providers, contacting them, and being put on waiting lists is another barrier to finding care. Work schedules, caregiving duties, and lack of access to a phone, a computer, and the internet all may complicate this process. Mental illness symptoms and disability also can make it challenging to find treatment when the process is usually complicated and involves a large time commitment. Some decide not to pursue treatment as a result, or they eventually give up after not being able to find a provider with an opening.

When outpatient treatment is not available, mental illness symptoms can become severe enough to require emergency intervention. In some cases outpatient treatment is not sufficient; however, more intensive inpatient treatment is also in low supply. In 2021 the Substance Abuse and Mental Health Services Administration reported that facilities and hospitals are at 144 percent capacity for inpatient beds for mental health care. For those requiring more specialized care, such as pediatric patients or those with severe mental illness or multiple diagnoses, accessing inpatient care can be even more challenging. The lack of facilities that can address individuals who are a safety risk or require more intensive treatment means that often these patients end up in hospital emergency rooms. Data from the National Hospital Ambulatory Medical Care Survey indi-

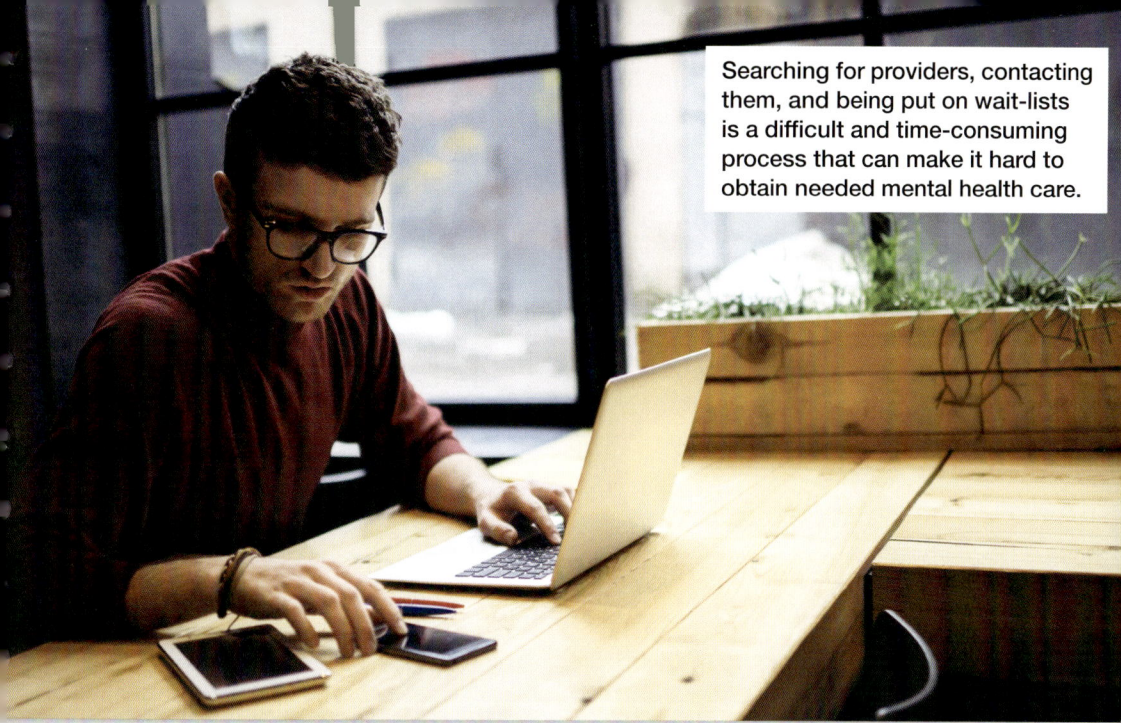

Searching for providers, contacting them, and being put on wait-lists is a difficult and time-consuming process that can make it hard to obtain needed mental health care.

cates that there has been an increase in mental health–related ER visits for pediatric patients. In 2011 there were 4.8 million mental health ER visits, representing 7.7 percent of all pediatric ER visits. In 2020 this had increased to 7.5 million, which accounted for 13.1 percent of all pediatric ER visits that year. Dr. Ryan Lawrence, director of the psychiatric emergency program at Columbia University Medical Center, says of this increase in ER visits:

> We are glad to see that people are looking for help. I hope it means there is less stigma and greater openness to getting connected to . . . mental health professionals. At the same time, if people are coming to the emergency room because they cannot get timely access to outpatient care, that's a problem that we all need to take seriously. . . . Some days there are multiple open beds and the wait time is short. At other times, it can take a few days for an inpatient psychiatry bed to become available. . . . While emergency room visits can be important in the short term, they are often a first step in a longer mental health journey.[20]

Financial Obstacles to Affordable Care

Although a shortage of mental health professionals is a barrier to accessing treatment, affordability is also a factor. Income levels and access to funds to pay for mental health services can deter people from seeking care, but so can complex and discriminatory governmental health care policies and the rising costs of insurance coverage. Even individuals who have health insurance may struggle to pay for mental health care. One issue is that health insurance companies handle mental health care differently than physical health care, and there are gaps in coverage as a result. Even as recently as the early 2000s, health insurance companies were not required to cover mental health expenses, and they relied on preexisting condition exclusions to deny coverage.

The Mental Health Parity and Addiction Equity Act of 2008 was passed to change this, yet progress toward obtaining more coverage for mental health services has been slow. Furthermore, federal agencies are still attempting to compel insurers to comply. Some insurance companies skirt the spirit of the law by vetoing prescribed medications or by limiting the number of days or sessions of a mental health service they will cover. The passage of the Affordable Care Act in 2010 enhanced both coverage and access, though the system is far from perfected.

Health insurance reimbursement to behavioral health providers is generally lower than to other medical professionals, especially primary care doctors, who mostly address physical maladies. A 2019 Milliman research report that analyzed the disparities between reimbursements found that primary care physicians were reimbursed 16.3 to 22.3 percent more than behavioral health providers. For example, an insurance company might reimburse a therapist $44 for a 50-minute therapy session, along with a $40 copay paid by the patient. A primary care physician might be reimbursed $95 plus a $20 copay paid by the patient for an appointment that may last only 15 or 30 minutes. Factoring in

Why Black Americans Often Turn Away from Professional Mental Health Assistance

"Stereotypes like . . . the 'strong black man,' and the 'strong black woman' are key examples of the over-saturation of black characteristics. . . . It is clear that when health is denied and disproportionately available, it disparages those who it discriminates against from seeking it. As the old adage says, 'when one door closes another one opens,' which is why many black people often turn to church instead of healthcare, where they often were ostracized. With black people being denied access to mental healthcare, it hinders them from seeking professional medical help, turning them to religion, and therefore causing black people to deny their mental and physical health in favor of church. The church has been one of the few places black people were able to release mental health concerns and crises, even though the results are not scientific, and do not include trained professionals or medication. This leads to things like generational trauma continuing through a cycle.

With more and more black people turning to therapy as a solution to their mental health issues, it opens a door to opportunity to heal old wounds, so someday things like generational trauma can be healed, and the cycle can be broken."

Award-winning essay by Kyle, a North Carolina teen

Kyle, "How the Neglect of Mental Health Within Black Communities Causes Underlying Issues," National Institute on Minority Health and Health Disparities, May 31, 2024. www.nimhd.nih.gov.

---

the time to file insurance claims, resolve denied claims, or speed delayed payments, it is not surprising that many mental health professionals no longer accept insurance. This drastic move is a means for professionals to curb burnout and preserve their own mental health, but it is also an attempt to give patients the care they need without having to prove to their health insurance provider that they need it.

Various studies and surveys have estimated that at least 30 to 45 percent of psychiatrists and therapists no longer accept insurance for these reasons. Similarly, patients with limited or no out-of-network coverage may have to pay completely out of

> "Insurance companies can be pretty hands on with their management. Some only authorize eight sessions at a time.... I think that the problems that we're grappling with here are just indicative of capitalism in general and a capitalist healthcare industry."[21]
>
> —Peter H. Addy, licensed professional counselor

pocket with no reimbursement for visit costs. An Access Across America report conducted by Milliman in 2021 found that the average cost of a psychotherapy session was $174. This is not sustainable for most Americans, especially when monthly or weekly sessions might be necessary for treatment.

Other loopholes that health insurance companies use to avoid covering mental health (and often other medical) treatment include requiring patients to pay high deductibles before the companies cover any additional costs or not considering certain mental health treatment "medically necessary." Peter H. Addy, a licensed professional counselor, says of the various roadblocks:

> Insurance companies can be pretty hands on with their management. Some only authorize eight sessions at a time. And then if you want to do another eight sessions, you'd have to reapply or they want to see a treatment plan or something like that.... I think that the problems that we're grappling with here are just indicative of capitalism in general and a capitalist healthcare industry.[21]

Populations with the Most Difficulties Accessing Care

While lack of working professionals and high financial costs of treatment are huge barriers, there are certain populations that acutely have trouble accessing treatment. Dr. Joshua Gordon recalls two different patients who had the same diagnosis but experienced disparities in receiving treatment. One was a Hispanic homeless man who arrived in the ER in a psychotic state and demanded medication that had been stolen from him. The other was a White woman he treated at his private practice. Her symptoms were well managed, and she arrived with records of her former treatment and in-depth knowledge of her diagnosis. Gordon reflects:

> Both patients were young adults. Both had severe bipolar disorder. Both had survived a suicide attempt. Their medication lists were the same. Their lives were not.
>
> Differences in health outcomes like these can reflect a number of underlying factors, including biological factors or environmental exposures; social, economic, and cultural contexts; and access to quality health care. When these differences adversely affect disadvantaged populations, they are known as health disparities.[22]

In this specific example, race, quality of treatment that the patient was able to afford, and housing were all factors in each patient's ability to obtain treatment, sustain the program, and continually access medication. Homeless individuals are one segment of the American population who find it increasingly difficult to treat their mental illness. Lack of financial resources, challenges in obtaining services, lack of a safe living situation, and high susceptibility to other illnesses can all aggravate mental illness symptoms.

Individuals of color also have increased difficulty accessing mental health treatment. Systemic racism has been part of the psychological field since its development over the past two centuries. For instance, psychology has been used to support eugenics theories, champion laws enforcing segregation and banning interracial marriage, and defend colonialist practices, such as government-sponsored boarding schools for Indigenous children and teens. Psychological research still underrepresents individuals of color in everything from population studies to the development of diagnostic tools. This leads to higher rates of misdiagnosis

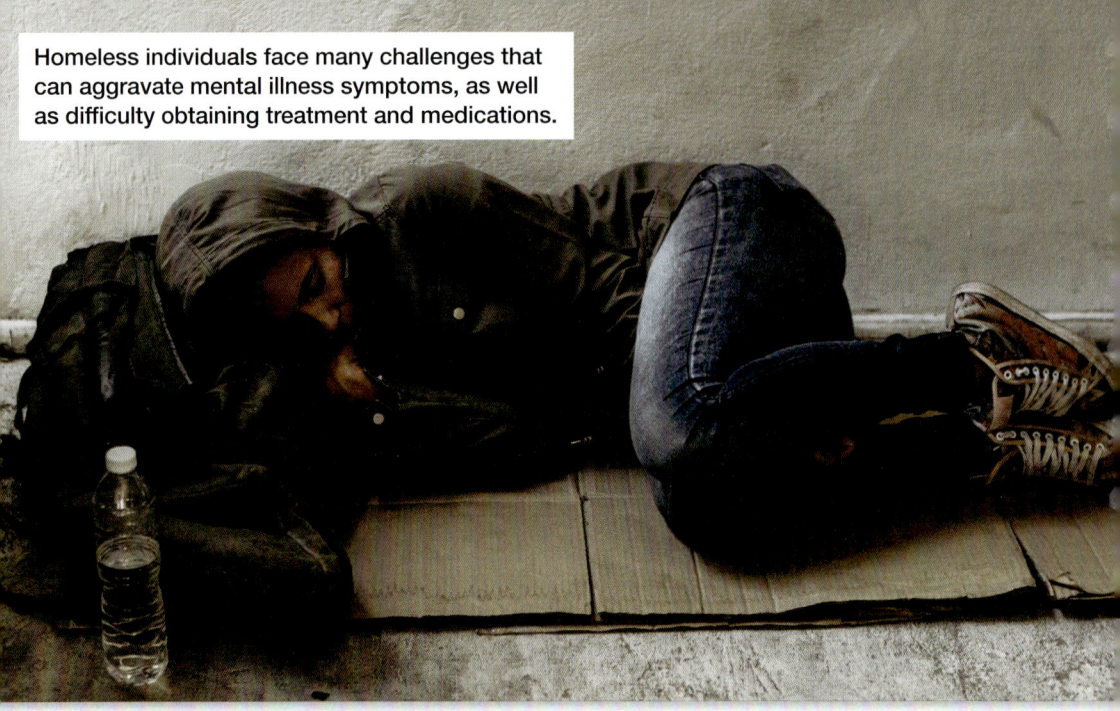

Homeless individuals face many challenges that can aggravate mental illness symptoms, as well as difficulty obtaining treatment and medications.

or late diagnosis for many children, teens, and adults of color. In 2021 the American Psychological Association released a resolution apologizing for its role in both promoting and perpetuating racism, discrimination, and the belief that certain races are biologically superior to others. The resolution stated:

> Since its origins as a scientific discipline in the mid-19th century, psychology has, through acts of commission and omission, contributed to the dispossession, displacement, and exploitation of communities of color. . . . Psychology has been complicit in failing to effectively elevate the science behind the disproportionate concentration of adverse social determinants of health in communities of color.[23]

With this history and emerging research that shows the impact of social factors and racism on people of color, it is not surprising that individuals within these groups often prefer to obtain treatment from doctors and therapists of color. However, these practitioners are even more difficult to find, since the majority of therapists, social workers, and doctors are White, and mental health professionals of color are also experiencing higher rates of burnout because they are in high demand.

Another historically marginalized community that experiences difficulties accessing treatment is the LGBTQ population. The discrimination, mistreatment, and isolation that LGBTQ individuals deal with on a daily basis means that they face higher rates of mental illness symptoms than the general population. A 2022 survey of thirty-four thousand LGBTQ young people aged thirteen to twenty-four found that 73 percent were experiencing symptoms of anxiety and 58 percent were experiencing symptoms of depression. Quality health care of all kinds can be difficult to come by for LGBTQ individuals, because many experience discrimination, judgment, and inferior medical treatment at the hands of biased health care professionals. Finding a therapist or doctor who is not only accepting and affirming of LGBTQ individuals but also well versed in challenges specific to their lives—so they feel safe and heard—can be extremely challenging.

Progress in Mental Health Care

While the barriers to accessing treatment can seem overwhelming or even insurmountable, health care policy nonprofits and government entities continue to fight for more equitable treatment for mental illnesses. One development arising from the COVID-19 pandemic was the expansion of commercial health insurance and Medicaid to cover telehealth visits. This has increased opportunities for individuals who may be unable to leave their home or do not have a provider nearby to see mental health providers who are licensed in their state. Hopefully, in the future there will be even more movement toward widening insurance coverage and increasing the pool of mental health professionals available to those in need of services.

CHAPTER THREE

Mental Illness and Violence

It is a common misconception that violence is a characteristic of mental illness. This belief is fed by the way mental illness is portrayed in movies, television, and even news media coverage of violent crime. Mental health professionals have long known that violence is not a symptom of mental illness, but mental illness might be one factor among many that induce individuals to act violently. Conversely, research has shown that the mentally ill are more likely to be victims rather than perpetrators of violence.

Links Between Violence and Mental Illness

"Mental health may have been a factor in fatal shooting of man's father, friend says," reads the headline of a February 16, 2022, article on a Spokane, Washington, news site. The article is an update on a previous news story reporting on a twenty-four-year-old man who contacted 911 after shooting his father in the head. A friend had recognized the man's declining mental health and suicidal thoughts and had previously tried to get him assistance. However, the article also reveals that this man had substance abuse issues and was on methamphetamine when he developed a plan for killing his father. These details are not the focus of the article, nor are they included in the headline.

Psychologists and psychiatrists have determined that violence itself is not a symptom of any mental illness. However, there are some mental illness symptoms that can result in some individuals being more prone to violence. The first of these are delusions, known as persecutory delusions, that result from paranoia. They lead an individual to believe that another person or persons are targeting them for harm. Command hallucinations can cause an individual to hear voices that are ordering them to do things, such as harm themselves or other people. These symptoms generally occur in mental illnesses known as psychotic disorders. Psychotic disorders include schizophrenia, schizoaffective disorder, and catatonia. Various studies have estimated that the prevalence of psychotic disorders in the United States is 0.25 to 0.64 percent of the population.

Psychosis as a symptom can also be a result of a brain tumor, head injury, Alzheimer's disease, stroke, Parkinson's disease, and substance abuse. Bipolar disorder, a mood disorder, can include psychosis as a symptom during periods of mania. A 2021 *Monitor on Psychology* article notes that people with bipolar disorder "can be overtaken by an exaggerated sense of their own power, which can stunt their ability to empathize with others and foster a sense of entitlement, including the right to take advantage of or exploit others. . . . Similarly, the high energy that often accompanies mania can lead to violence or aggression on its own terms."[24] The National Institute of Mental Health estimates that 2.6 percent of Americans have been diagnosed with bipolar disorder.

Another possible mental health connection is with symptoms of personality disorders such as adolescent conduct disorder and antisocial personality disorder. Antisocial personality disorder's hallmark symptoms include deceit and manipulation of others, disregard of others and societal expectations and laws, lack of remorse or responsibility for one's actions, and anger and hostility that can lead to physical aggression. A 2016 research article using data from the MacArthur Violence Risk Assessment Study identified one hundred former inpatients with repeat episodes of violence and determined that only 12 percent of them had experienced an episode of psychosis prior to the violent act. However, all one hundred individuals met the criteria for antisocial personality disorder and had a history of uncontrolled anger and conduct issues. The American Psychiatric Association estimates that antisocial personality disorder impacts 0.6 to 3.6 percent of Americans.

Most targeted studies and research over the past few decades on potential links between mental illness and violence have revealed no strong connection. A variety of studies have found that only 1 percent of violent offenders have a diagnosed mental illness, and only 3 to 5 percent of violent acts are committed by

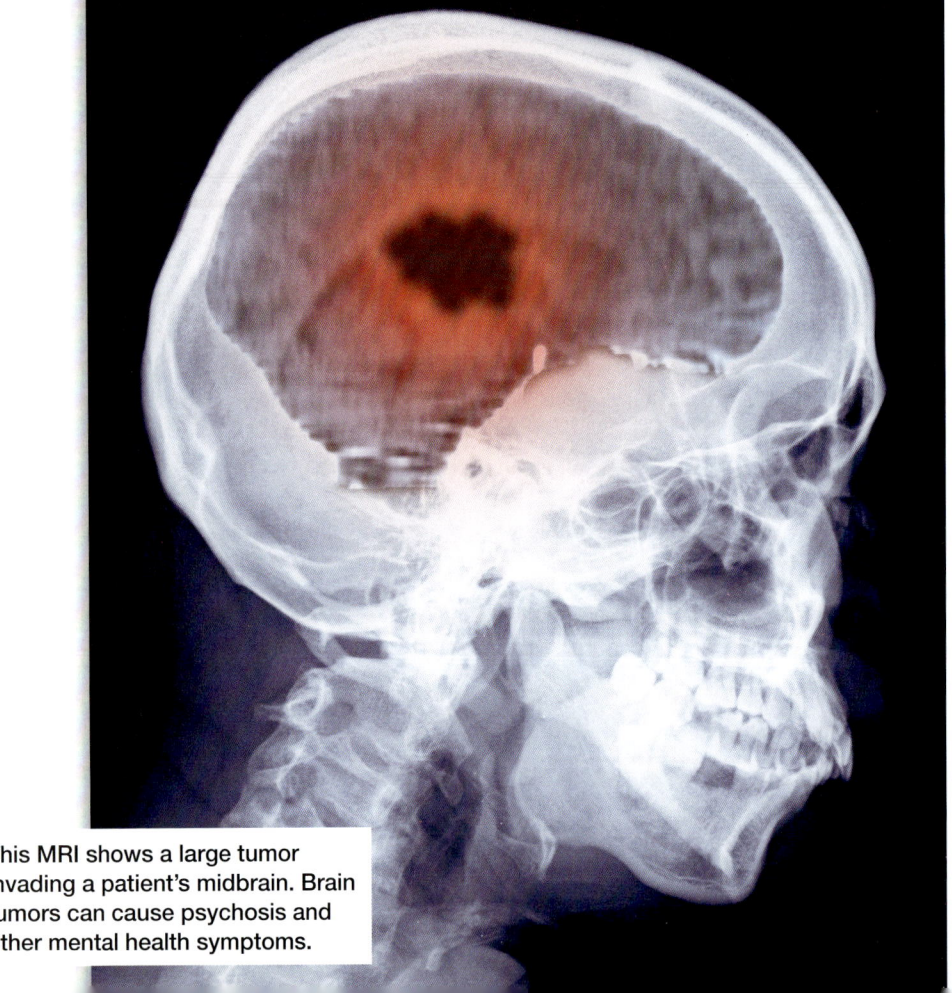

This MRI shows a large tumor invading a patient's midbrain. Brain tumors can cause psychosis and other mental health symptoms.

an individual with a mental illness. A research team visited one American community and administered an aggressiveness questionnaire to 121 individuals, some of whom had mental illness diagnoses. The researchers published their findings in a 2020 edition of *New Ideas in Psychology*:

> The results revealed that there is no statistically significant difference in terms of violence and crime involvement between individuals with a mental health diagnosis and those without. Moreover, the study did not find any statistically significant associations between specific mental health disorders and specific crime offences. The findings suggest that certain mental health disorders do not strongly contribute to crime violence and involvement.[25]

The choice to conduct this specific study with a community sample was intentional. Many former studies had surveyed only high-risk individuals such as prison inmates or psychiatric patients, who did not represent the broader community. While the authors of this research report question whether the relationship between violence and mental illness has been significantly overestimated, even among the potentially biased surveys that came before, the correlation between mental illness and violence was statistically small.

Researchers acknowledge that correlation does not equal causation, especially when there are many other factors that could impact a tendency for violence. These factors exist across populations as well as among those who have been diagnosed with a mental illness. A 2012 study looked at the 34,653 people from the 2001–2005 National Epidemiologic Survey on Alcohol

> "There is no statistically significant difference in terms of violence and crime involvement between individuals with a mental health diagnosis and those without."[25]
>
> —Research published in 2020 in *New Ideas in Psychology*

and Related Conditions. The findings showed that in the two to four years since the original data was collected, 2.9 percent of individuals with serious mental illness had committed a violent act, compared with 0.8 percent of those who had neither a serious mental illness nor a substance abuse disorder. A study published in 2019 by researchers at Yale University and East Tennessee State University added new insight on the topic of mental illness and violence. The study found that the individuals surveyed who had substance abuse disorders, especially drug users, or both substance abuse disorders and mental health disorders were the ones most at risk of committing a violent crime or becoming incarcerated.

However, as Eric B. Elbogen, a psychologist who studies violence and mental illness, says, "If a person has a severe mental illness, [they] may have other risk factors for violent behavior. So, it may not be mental illness that is driving the violence at all, but rather factors like having been abused as a child, being unemployed, or living in a high-crime neighborhood."[26] Other risk factors for violent behavior that have been identified are personal crises such as divorce, job loss or other financial crisis, and being the victim of a crime or victim of abuse. Additional impacts on future violent behavior include adverse experiences during childhood such as abuse or neglect and housing or food insecurity.

A Flawed but Popular Perception

Although a very small percentage of the mentally ill population is responsible for violent behavior and crime, the public narrative often runs counter to the facts. The responsibility for that prevailing narrative lies in part with the news media and their reporting on crime and mental illness. This includes presenting biased or inaccurate coverage, attributing crimes to mental illness without verifying diagnosis, and not consulting expert sources for coverage of crimes. Media coverage on mental illness tends to focus

How to Fact-Check Media Coverage

When reading media coverage about mental illness (or any topic), fact-checking is important to ensure that the information provided is accurate. Here are some questions to consider:

- What outlet is providing the story? Is it a reputable news outlet? What is the political leaning of the outlet, and could this have affected how the story was covered?

- Is the headline written to encourage clicks (online) or to keep people reading or watching? Is it misleading?

- Have experts been consulted to offer perspective? If so, who are they and what is their background?

- If this is an opinion piece, what is the background of the journalist or writer? What in the author's background or experience could introduce bias?

- If anyone is identified as having a mental illness, has a diagnosis been verified, or is the claim based on the opinions of friends, family members, or other nonexpert observers?

- If sources such as studies or other articles are referenced, do they only reference the parts that support the argument, ignoring the scope of the original?

largely on incidents in which a history of mental illness is brought up in the description of a violent criminal. Often, no other potential contributing factors are mentioned or highlighted. As in the case of the young man who killed his father likely while under the influence of drugs, inflammatory and misleading headlines also can color public perceptions, especially if all that people read is a headline.

Studies of news media representation of mental illness support this conclusion. A 2017 study conducted by Marian Chen and Stephen Lawrie identified two hundred articles featuring mental health over a four-week period from nine UK daily newspapers and discovered that over half of the articles had a negative tone and 18.5 percent were associated with violence. A similar Canadian study that analyzed television news coverage from

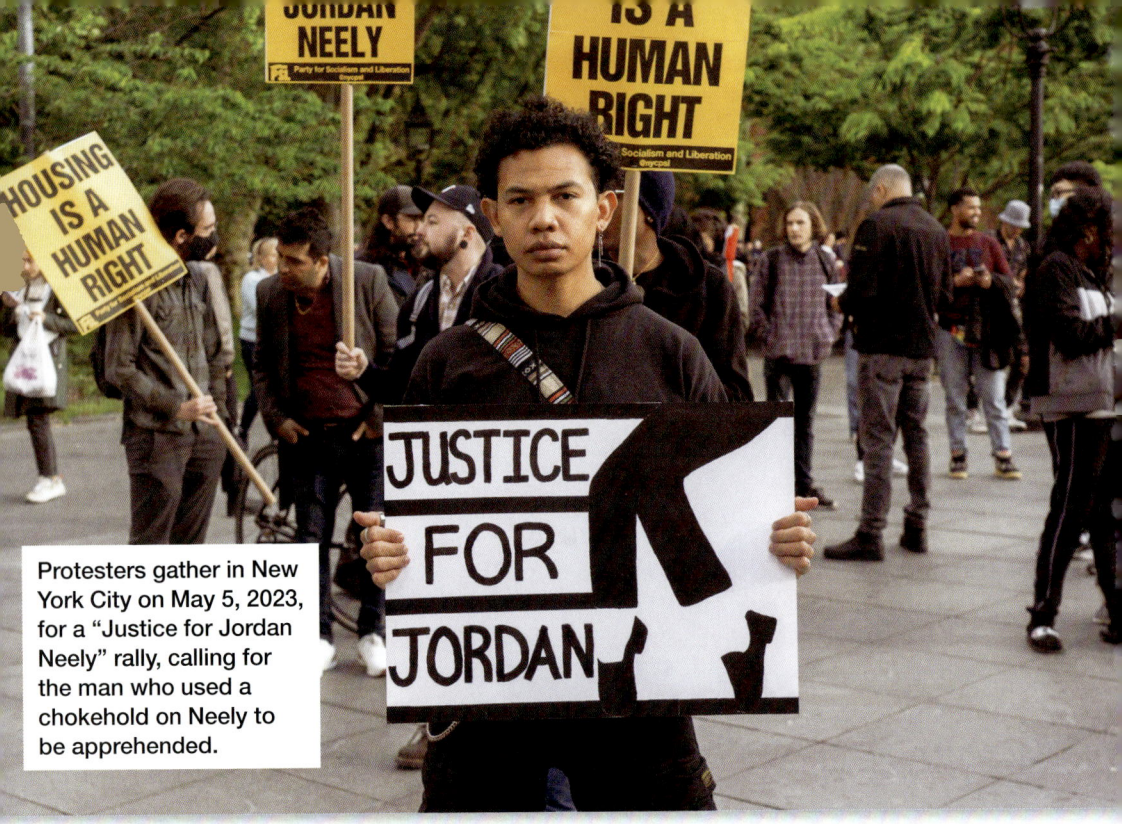

Protesters gather in New York City on May 5, 2023, for a "Justice for Jordan Neely" rally, calling for the man who used a chokehold on Neely to be apprehended.

2013 to 2015 found that in 2015, 60 percent of coverage had a negative tone and over 50 percent of the news clips connected mental illness with violence. Often, the same events can result in stories that come to very different conclusions about mental illness and violence. For example, Freddie deBoer's *New York* op-ed "The Case for Forcing the Mentally Ill into Treatment" uses the tragic murder of mentally ill Jordan Neely by Daniel Penny as support for his argument. Witnesses testified that Neely, who was Black and homeless, was shouting but not acting violently when Penny, a Marine, placed Neely into a chokehold that ended his life on a New York City subway. In the editorial, DeBoer claims, "If we care enough for Neely to imagine a world in which he would have survived, then we almost certainly must imagine one in which he was forced into care. . . . I argued last year that involuntary treatment could have saved his life."[27] Conversely, Olayemi Olurin's piece in *Teen Vogue* uses Neely's case to focus on the fact that he was the victim of manslaughter. She writes:

Daniel Penny got to go home after killing Jordan Neely and it took days for the district attorney's office to announce that he'd be charged with second-degree manslaughter. Meanwhile, right after the killing, the press quickly released the unrelated rap sheet of the victim. And I could launch into an explanation of why Neely's rap sheet is not proof of criminality nor should it condemn him to death. . . . But I won't get into that because no matter how many people want to pretend otherwise, Neely is not on trial. He's dead.[28]

Researchers have found that stigmas surrounding mental illness and violence have increased over the years. In a 2019 study published in *Health Affairs*, researchers studied trends in the National Stigma Survey from 1996, 2006, and 2018 and found that support had increased over 10 percent for forced hospitalization for those with schizophrenia. Twenty percent of respondents in 2018 also believed that legal force should be used to put those with "daily troubles"—which was defined as feeling sad, being worried, and having trouble sleeping, rather than any strict mental illness diagnosis—into a psychiatric hospital. "What it tells me is that right now we're living in a very fearful society. The myth of dangerousness is deep in our culture," the study's author Bernice Pescosolido says. "But 'sick' does not mean mentally ill. It's sort of our American metaphor for anybody who is outside the norm."[29]

Media coverage of mental illness is also typically sensationalized to encourage readers and viewers to read news stories or continue to watch video programming. There is also a tendency for individuals to be drawn to and remember information that confirms their beliefs about a certain topic. This is known as confirmation bias. When celebrities or political figures share inaccurate information in a public forum or a news article, those who admire and trust them are likely to believe what they say. Donald Trump, for example, has blamed school shootings on mental illness on multiple occasions, contributing to the rhetoric that mental illness is the trigger for violence. Often, both news coverage and individual perception that violence is a result of mental illness springs from a desire to explain why people do horrible things to each other. Psychology researchers Sherry Glied and Richard G. Frank assert, "When a horrific and inexplicable act of violence occurs . . . people, quite reasonably, recognize the perpetrator's behavior as abnormal. Journalists, investigating the story, seek and frequently find long-standing symptoms of a mental disorder: the perpetrator had been depressed, was a loner, or had sought treatment of a mental health problem."[30] But Glied and Frank fear that even though the link between mental illness and violence is weak at best, the reporting and implication of a connection only further stigmatizes all those who suffer from such illnesses.

The Mentally Ill as Victims of Violence

Those studying the connections between mental illness and violence have discovered that the mentally ill are more likely to be victims than perpetrators of violence. This victimization has a centuries-long history. For many years those who were institutionalized were abused by staff members and subjected to treatments that were traumatic and would be considered torture by modern standards. People with mental illness are still subject to abuses and physical and sexual violence while in outpatient and inpatient treatment. A 2020 study of 170 individuals with severe mental illness found that 30.6 percent had been raped and 64.7 percent had been the victim of physical violence with or without a weapon outside of the mental health care system. Inside the mental health system, they also experienced violence. Some of this violence involved staff members: 10.6 percent reported physical violence and 3.5 percent reported sexual assault by staff. Some of this violence involved fellow patients: 17.1 percent had experienced physical violence and 7.1 percent had experienced sexual assault

Mental Health Crisis Teams

In most areas of the country, police are the first responders to mental health crises. This has led to the death, injury, and forceful detainment of many individuals with mental illness. In most cases the police are simply not trained to address mental health crises and can often escalate situations rather than de-escalate them. Even the presence of an armed police officer can result in fearful or impulsive decisions that can lead a resolvable situation to go awry. Some cities have begun to implement crisis teams with trained professionals to address nonviolent mental health or substance abuse–related incidents. These teams are made up of professionals such as emergency medical technicians, therapists, social workers, and sometimes even peer specialists who have experienced mental illness and can help build rapport with the individuals assisted. Another key feature of these programs is connecting those struggling to the right resources, such as food, medical treatment, or follow-up mental health care. When Denver, Colorado, implemented its Support Team Assisted Response program in 2020, in the first six months specialists were able to resolve 748 mental health calls without any force being used or arrests being made.

by other patients. Further, 37.6 percent had been put in restraints and 25.9 percent had been strip-searched by staff.

It is estimated that the mentally ill experience violence at ten to eleven times the frequency of the general population. A 2014 research study by Sarah Desmarais and others found that 30.9 percent of their database of 4,480 adults with mental illness had experienced violence in the previous six months, 43.7 percent of these more than once. The research also revealed that 23.9 percent of those studied had committed a violent act, but they were eleven times more likely to have been the victims of violence previously. Desmarais says:

> This highlights the need for more robust public health interventions that are focused on violence. It shouldn't just be about preventing adults with mental illness from committing violent acts, it should also be about protecting those at risk of being victimized. . . .

While correlation is not necessarily causation, preventing violence against the mentally ill may drive down instances of violence committed by the mentally ill.[31]

> "While correlation is not necessarily causation, preventing violence against the mentally ill may drive down instances of violence committed by the mentally ill."[31]
>
> —Sarah Desmarais, psychology researcher

Beyond being victimized by patients and staff at mental health care facilities and being more vulnerable to violence while out in the world, the mentally ill are also at risk of victimization by the police. The *Washington Post* tracks fatal shootings involving police and has found that from 2015 to October 2024, 20 percent of the victims, or two thousand individuals, were shot and killed while in the midst of a mental health crisis. Violent policing in response to individuals deemed a threat, especially those individuals who are experiencing a mental health crisis, calls for both police reforms and interventions by trained crisis teams instead of police.

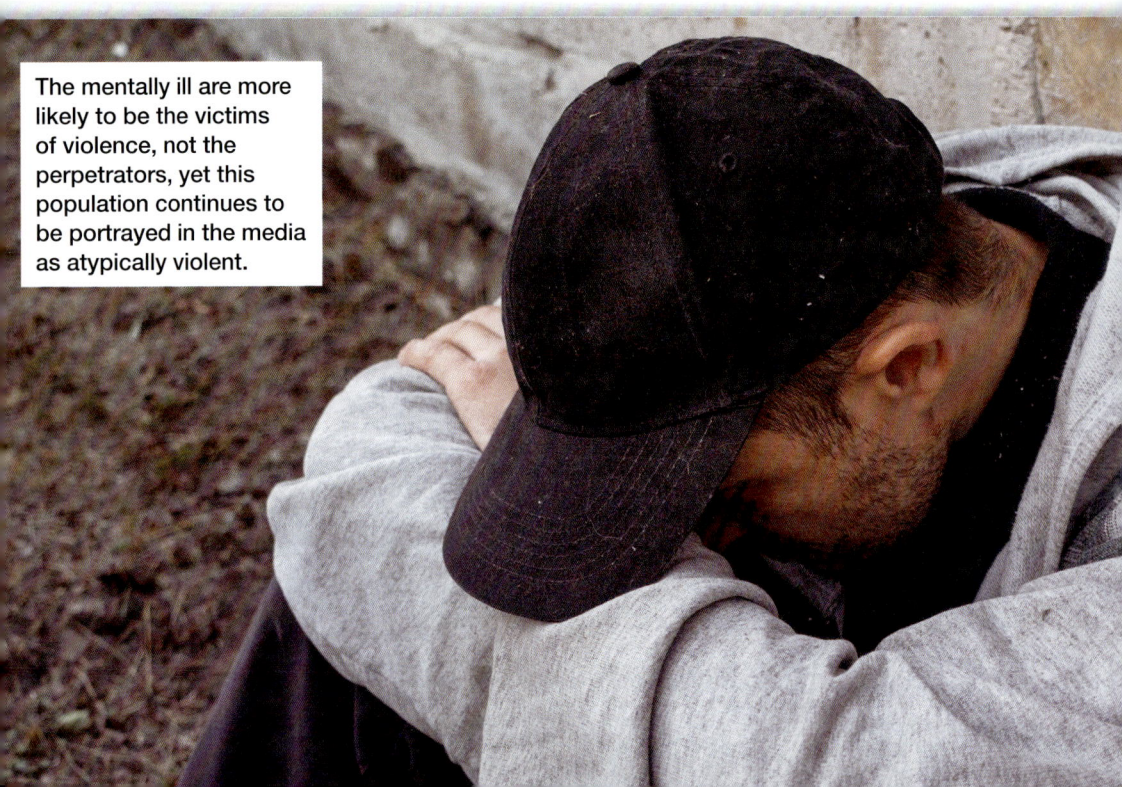

The mentally ill are more likely to be the victims of violence, not the perpetrators, yet this population continues to be portrayed in the media as atypically violent.

Protections for the Mentally Ill

Despite media coverage and flawed studies, the mentally ill are actually responsible for only a small percentage of violent crime. Yet the mentally ill population continues to be portrayed as atypically violent. The American Psychological Association and other interest groups hope to counter this stereotype so that violent crime is not automatically linked to mental illness. Instead, more research is needed into the other factors within America's communities that may contribute to violence. Reshaping the rhetoric will require reforms that promote mental health care and counteract erroneous messaging about mental illness and the mentally ill.

CHAPTER FOUR

Mental Illness and Homelessness

It is estimated that approximately 20 to 30 percent of the homeless population suffer from severe mental illness. The homeless population is often dehumanized, viewed as a collective problem or unsightly stain on cities rather than as individuals who are suffering. This has led to recent efforts to criminalize homelessness, an effort to remove the problem from city streets rather than providing needed services to homeless individuals. Thus, those who suffer both homelessness and mental illness are often doubly stigmatized in society.

Rates of Mental Illness Among the Homeless

Not unlike violence and mental illness, the connection between homelessness and mental illness has been studied by psychologists for some time. The results of this research have been more conclusive, indicating that a significant segment of the homeless population suffers from mental illness, but that mental illness is not a cause of homelessness. The 2023 US Department of Housing and Urban Development (HUD) Continuum of Care homelessness assessment report found that out of 653,104 homeless individuals it had identified, 20.9 percent had severe mental illness and 16.5 percent struggled with chronic substance abuse. A 2021 review by Stefan Gutwinski and Stefanie Schreiter of thirty-nine studies from eleven higher-income countries found that there was an average of 76.2 percent of individuals with mental disorders among the eight thousand homeless individuals studied. This included 36.7 percent with alcohol abuse disorders, 12.4 percent with schizophrenia spectrum disorders, and 12.6 percent with major depression. Other studies have estimated that 20 to 30 percent of the homeless population have serious mental illnesses such as major depression, bipolar disorder, and schizophrenia. This also means that the majority of those who are homeless are not experiencing severe mental illness, although this has become a stereotype about the homeless population.

Impact of Unemployment on Homelessness

Unemployment is one of the top causes of homelessness, along with a lack of affordable housing and health care and stagnant wages. A 2019 Charles Schwab modern wealth survey determined that 59 percent of Americans live paycheck to paycheck. This means that a job loss could very well leave average Americans unable to pay their rent or mortgage and soon without a home. Since 2020, unemployment, inflation, and housing costs have all risen. Unsurprisingly, so has the number of homeless Americans. HUD determined that the number of homeless individuals had increased by 12 percent, or 70,650 people, from 2022 to 2023, and since 2019 it has grown by 23.3 percent. Resources and shelters for homeless individuals have simply not been able to keep up with the demand. Not all homeless individuals have diagnosed mental illness or have had mental illness symptoms prior to becoming homeless. However, the strain of being homeless can often lead to experiencing them. Breaktime, a Boston nonprofit that serves homeless young adults, says:

> People experiencing homelessness endure great amounts of stress, which can cause increased anxiety, fear, insomnia, depression, paranoia, and substance use. . . . People

experiencing homelessness . . . face constant threats—from daily survival needs and inhospitable living conditions to crime and violence—and the resulting chronic stress can be debilitating and overwhelming, negatively impacting mental and physical health over time.[32]

Those who were mentally ill prior to becoming homeless are also impacted by this consistent stress, which can increase symptoms and the likelihood of them remaining homeless for longer periods. Financial means certainly have an impact on this because people who cannot afford to house and feed themselves also cannot afford treatment or medication.

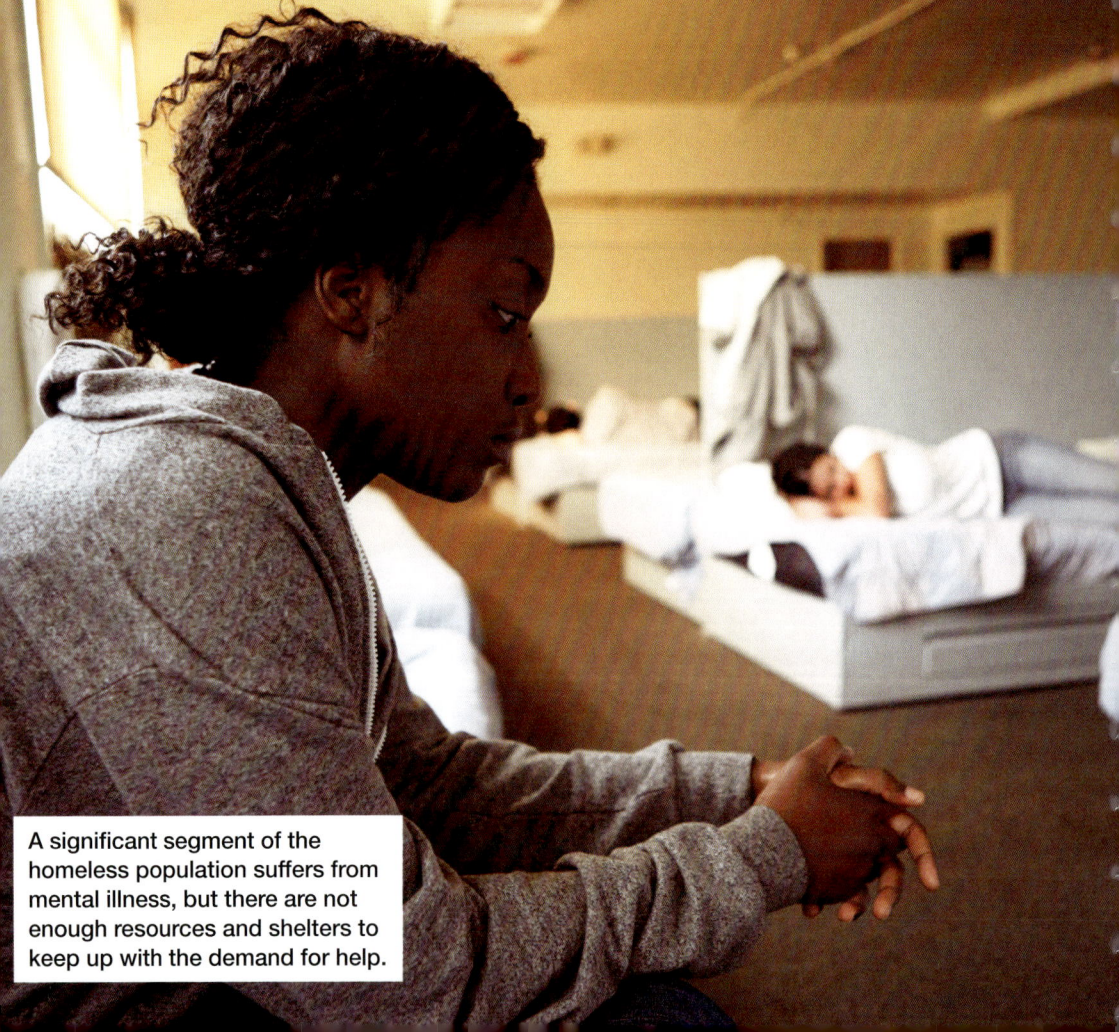

A significant segment of the homeless population suffers from mental illness, but there are not enough resources and shelters to keep up with the demand for help.

Those with severe mental illness are at risk for higher rates of unemployment. Those diagnosed with schizophrenia and other psychotic disorders especially have difficulties obtaining and maintaining employment. Various studies estimate that 70 to 90 percent of those with schizophrenia are unemployed, even though up to 90 percent want paid employment. The 2016 *Global Burden of Diseases, Injuries, and Risk Factors Study* found that schizophrenia was the number fifteen global cause of disability, which is significant due to the small portion of the population it affects. High rates of unemployment are due not just to individuals being unable to work but also to employer discrimination.

A study published in the *Australian Journal of Psychiatry* in 2018 examined negative stereotypes about psychosis and individuals' ability to maintain employment by interviewing patients, health care professionals, employers, and community members. Many assumed that those with psychosis could not work, could only work part time, did not want to work, could only do low-stress or menial jobs, or could be a liability to employers. Anecdotal accounts gathered from focus groups found that these stereotypes were in most cases false but persisted in the medical community and in the workplace. One individual with schizophrenia reflected, "I know people who hear voices or receive messages in their heads and I know that they're capable of working and for some reason they've been put on the scrapheaps for the rest of their lives. It's an extremely serious problem." Another individual with bipolar disorder believes that she is more at risk when she is unemployed, saying, "When I'm in work I'm on top of the world. I have a lot going for me, I can see a future. . . , I can see myself doing a lot of things. If I'm unemployed. . . , I don't see any kind

> "People experiencing homelessness . . . face constant threats—from daily survival needs and inhospitable living conditions to crime and violence—and the resulting chronic stress can be debilitating and overwhelming."[32]
>
> —Breaktime, a Boston nonprofit

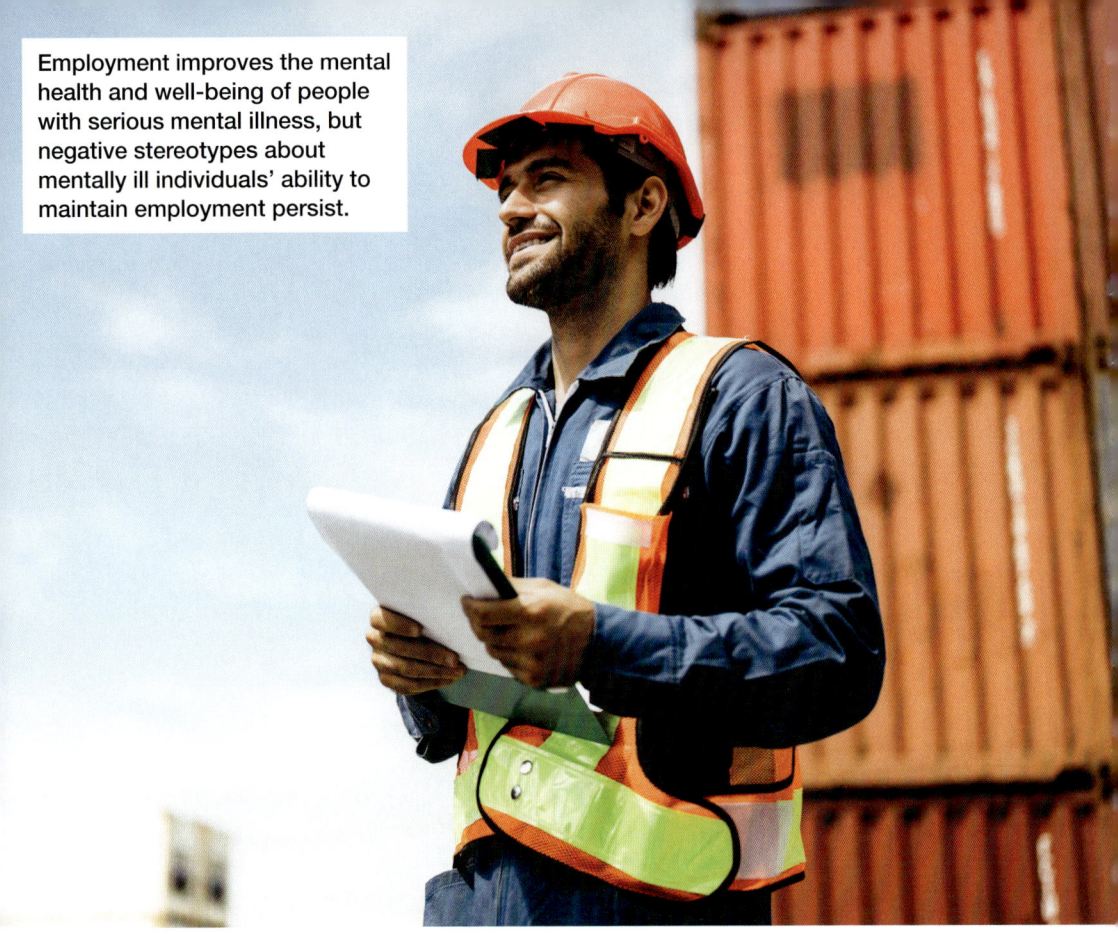

Employment improves the mental health and well-being of people with serious mental illness, but negative stereotypes about mentally ill individuals' ability to maintain employment persist.

of a future or anything for myself . . . nothing . . . may as well not even be alive."[33] This connection between employment and better outcomes for those with mental illness has been recognized by the psychiatric community as well. A 2020 *Epidemiology and Psychiatric Sciences* editorial declared the following:

> Employment improves the mental health and wellbeing of people with serious mental disorders, including improved self-esteem, symptom control, quality of life, social relationships and community integration, without harmful side effects. . . . Employment engenders self-reliance and leads to other valued outcomes, including self-confidence, the respect of others, personal income and community integration.[34]

Severe Mental Illness and Homelessness

Beyond the impact of severe mental illness on being able to secure and maintain employment that is full time and not low paid, symptoms of mental illnesses such as schizophrenia can also impact whether individuals end up homeless and stay homeless. Symptoms such as psychosis can lead to individuals experiencing hallucinations and delusions. These often can lead sufferers to feel distrustful of others or unsafe or persecuted in and out of the workplace. Symptoms of social withdrawal might also contribute to a desire to isolate from others, even those who may be trying to help, such as friends or family members. Medication for mental illnesses such as bipolar disorder and schizophrenia is key to treatment and reduction of symptoms, but individuals with these disorders may either refuse to take medication entirely or not take it as prescribed. Side effects, lack of access, and forgetfulness may hamper the regular taking of medication, but often patients either believe they do not need the medication because they are not sick or they stop taking it after their symptoms improve. One symptom of schizophrenia is anosognosia, or a lack of understanding that one has an illness, caused by impairment to thought processes. Paranoia and delusions can also lead individuals with schizophrenia to believe that their medication is causing their psychosis or that it is harming them in some other way.

Some individuals with psychosis, and even those who are not experiencing it, may also feel safer outdoors than in workplaces or crowded shelters or other housing. Shelters are not always safe environments for homeless individuals, especially those who have experienced prior trauma or have difficulty trusting others. Shelters also have many rules that may mean being separated from a pet, belongings, or a partner; being subject to a curfew; and having to leave during the day. Esperanza Fonseca, who has been homeless in California, reported of her time in a shelter, "The most painful thing was to watch women leave the shelter to go back to the streets because they thought it was better. . . . In the shelter, I was subjected to violence, threats, harassment, discrimination. That is what we feared we would face in the streets, but we still experienced it at the shelter, just with more rules and expired milk."[35] In many locations, there are limited routes for obtaining permanent private housing, or more permanent housing is offered only with prerequisites or conditions that disqualify those with mental illness or substance abuse disorders. And lack of a permanent address can make it difficult to find or hold a job.

> "In the shelter, I was subjected to violence, threats, harassment, discrimination. That is what we feared we would face in the streets, but we still experienced it at the shelter, just with more rules and expired milk."[35]
>
> —Esperanza Fonseca, a homeless individual

Ashley Womble's brother became homeless after he had been recently diagnosed with schizophrenia and refused to take medication. He was experiencing hallucinations and believed that the government was surveilling him. Womble reflects, "With everything going on inside his mind, he did not want to be inside himself. He wanted to be able to move, to walk or hitchhike, and talk to strangers he met along the way." He traveled to the West Coast, where he was able to feel a sort of safety and security. Womble remembers speaking to him about California: "He reported that the weather was great and you could sleep in the parks. Whether or not you could sleep in the park and if the library was open 24/7 were major amenities to him. He was thrilled that there were so many people that would listen to him talk about his belief that the world would be ending very soon."[36]

Efforts to Solve the "Homeless Problem"

On June 28, 2024, the Supreme Court ruled that in California and eight other western states, it is legal for authorities to punish

Being Homeless with Schizophrenia

"For me, becoming homeless was a direct result of schizophrenia. Because of the illness, I could not work the easiest job or focus enough to take even one class. The illness brought on a paranoia which led me to cut off all my family members and my closest friends. . . . Looking back, I clearly realize that by interpreting the world through the prism of untreated schizophrenia, my deepest desire was to remain detached from reality. Caught in a world of delusion, my expectations were to become a world famous and powerful prophet and send billions of dollars of aid to people throughout the world who subsisted in poverty. . . . It would be three long years . . . until the time I was finally hospitalized. I was diagnosed with schizophrenia and antipsychotic medication was prescribed, (I wish it had been sooner). . . . But when the medication's severe side effects began to affect my everyday life, I discontinued my medication. . . . After gaining a deeper understanding of my diagnoses and the prospects for recovery, I restarted my medication and since then, have never missed a dose. . . . I am grateful for antipsychotic medication that has enabled me to reclaim a healthy mind and live with contentment in reality. I finished college and have found purposeful employment."

—Bethany Yeiser, woman with schizophrenia

Bethany Yeiser, "Schizophrenia and Homelessness: Paranoia Drove Me to Sleep Outside," *Recovery Road* (blog), *Psychology Today*, July 20, 2018. www.psychologytoday.com.

homeless individuals for sleeping outside. This criminalization of homelessness is one of the latest in efforts to address Americans' concerns about the growing homeless population. However, many cities already had anti-homeless laws in place that allow police to arrest individuals for loitering in a public place. In addition, actions such as living in vehicles, panhandling, sleeping in public locations, and even giving food to homeless individuals are illegal in various communities. Increases in the number of homeless individuals and the appearance of more homeless encampments since 2020 have made homelessness an even more visible problem, and one that many Americans prefer not to see. Homeless individuals are viewed as unhygienic, a public health risk, dangerous, mentally ill, and violent. When viewed through this lens, they are a problem to be fixed or removed, not human beings in need of assistance.

In late 2022 New York City mayor Eric Adams announced a policy that would make it easier to forcibly hospitalize homeless individuals that appear to be mentally ill. Journalist Caroline Lewis says of this effort:

> Mayor Adams has really been on this kick throughout his tenure in office so far of trying to target people who are street homeless or stay in the subways. . . . He's framed this as a way of helping New Yorkers feel safe. . . . He's been sending teams of clinicians and police officers to do outreach to people in the subways—both offering them services, but also just trying to get them to move somewhere else.[37]

Other cities are using similar tactics to remove homeless individuals from the streets. Advocates for the homeless believe measures like those proposed in New York City and similar measures

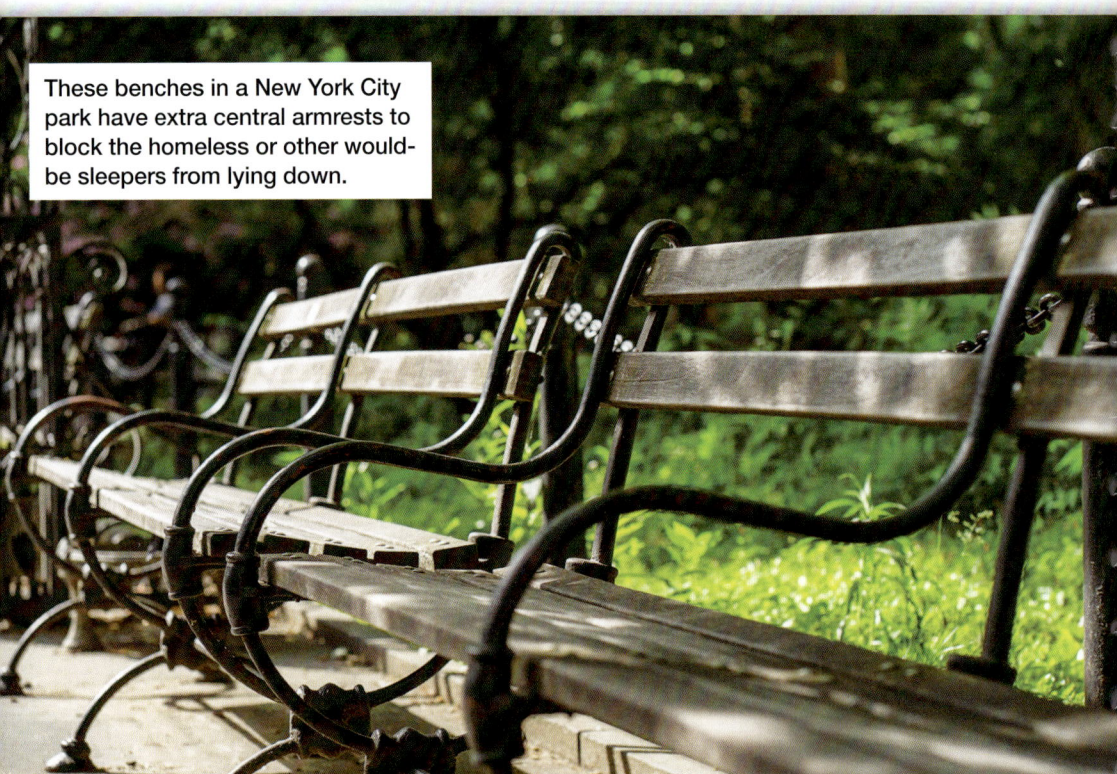

These benches in a New York City park have extra central armrests to block the homeless or other would-be sleepers from lying down.

Houston's Success at Addressing Homelessness

Most cities have a haphazard approach to addressing homelessness, leading to many people falling through the cracks. Beginning in 2011, Houston, Texas, began a concentrated effort to reduce homelessness in the city by uniting the organizations that serve this population. Now city agencies and over one hundred nonprofits coordinate services, which has reduced wasted time and allowed more individuals to be served. In 2011 Houston had the sixth-highest homeless population in the country, but by 2023 the number of homeless individuals in the city had been reduced by 64 percent. Houston has embraced a Housing First approach, which means individuals do not have to enter treatment before being able to obtain permanent housing. After housing is provided, individuals are connected with other resources, such as medical, addiction, and mental health treatment. Mandy Chapman Semple, who played a key part in developing Houston's new plan to address homelessness, says, "Our natural instinct when we see homelessness increasing is to hire more outreach workers and to build more shelter beds. The idea that if you have no permanent place to live, that you're also going to be able to transform and tackle complex mental health issues, addiction issues, complex financial issues? It's just unrealistic."

Quoted in Martha Teichner, "Inside Houston's Successful Strategy to Reduce Homelessness," CBS News, April 14, 2024. www.cbsnews.com.

being proposed in California and Oregon may violate civil rights. Opponents of forcible hospitalization are concerned about a return to an age when individuals could be institutionalized against their will and without cause. "Half a century ago . . . policymakers shuttered state psychiatric institutions, denouncing them as inhumane," NPR reports. "Involuntary commitment was deemphasized and state laws ensured that it only be used as a last resort. The thinking was that the patient should have autonomy and participate in their care."[38] Proponents argue that involuntary commitment is actually compassionate and gives mentally ill homeless individuals the right to medical care and, by extension, a better life.

Homelessness, however, is a complex issue, compounded by high housing costs, unemployment, and discrimination against both those in poverty and those experiencing mental illness. Advocates assert that addressing mental illness in the homeless population requires structural changes to achieve more affordable and accessible housing and health care, as well as access to jobs. They add that success in reducing the homeless population by providing safe, permanent housing coupled with needed health care work more effectively than efforts to criminalize homelessness or force individuals to be hospitalized.

SOURCE NOTES

Introduction: Mental Illness Beyond the Numbers

1. Quoted in Susan Shain and Aidan Gardiner, "30 People Tell Us What Homelessness Is Really Like," *New York Times*, March 6, 2023. www.nytimes.com.
2. Quoted in Shain and Gardiner, "30 People Tell Us What Homelessness Is Really Like."
3. Sarah Erdreich, "Last Fall, I Walked into a Psych Ward and Asked to Be Locked In. It Was Nothing like I Expected," *Slate*, March 11, 2022. https://slate.com.
4. Quoted in Young Invincibles, "Invincible Voices—Young Adult Mental Health Stories from Across the Nation," November 23, 2023. https://younginvincibles.org.

Chapter One: Misunderstanding Mental Illness

5. Putri Surya, "Please Don't Tell Me to Pray My Anxiety Away," Anxiety & Depression Association of America, August 23, 2018. https://adaa.org.
6. Surya, "Please Don't Tell Me to Pray My Anxiety Away."
7. American Psychiatric Association, "What Is Mental Illness?," 2022. www.psychiatry.org.
8. Substance Abuse and Mental Health Services Administration, *Key Substance Use and Mental Health Indicators in the United States: Results from the 2023 National Survey on Drug Use and Health*. Rockville, MD: Substance Abuse and Mental Health Services Administration, 2024. www.samhsa.gov.
9. Hara Estroff Marano, "Personal and Family History Are Important Information in Diagnosis," *The Therapy Center* (blog), *Psychology Today*, August 7, 2023. www.psychologytoday.com.
10. Quoted in Lynne Malcolm and Clare Blumer, "Madness and Insanity: A History of Mental Illness from Evil Spirits to Modern Medicine," ABC News, August 2, 2016. www.abc.net.au.
11. Tim Newman, "Medical Myths: Mental Health Misconceptions," Medical News Today, October 5, 2020. www.abc.net.au.
12. American Psychological Association, "What Psychological Factors Make People Susceptible to Believe and Act on Misinformation?," March 1, 2024. www.apa.org.
13. Kirsten Weir, "This Election Year, Fighting Misinformation Is Messier and More Important than Ever," *Monitor on Psychology*, January 1, 2024. www.apa.org.

14. Quoted in Julie Wood, "Managing Mental Health Misinformation on Social Media," Penn Medicine News, October 28, 2021. www.pennmedicine.org.
15. Quoted in Ellen McVay, "Social Media and Self-Diagnosis," Johns Hopkins Medicine, August 31, 2023. www.hopkinsmedicine.org.
16. Veronica Karp, "Doctors Reinforcing Mental Health Stigmas," Columbia University Mailman School of Public Health, October 3, 2022. www.publichealth.columbia.edu.

Chapter Two: The Challenges of Getting Care

17. Quoted in Jed Gottlieb, "An Era Where It Has Never Not Been About Drugs," *Harvard Gazette*, November 9, 2023. https://news.harvard.edu.
18. Pim Cuijpers et al., "A Network Meta-analysis of the Effects of Psychotherapies, Pharmacotherapies and Their Combination in the Treatment of Adult Depression," *World Psychiatry*, January 10, 2020. https://onlinelibrary.wiley.com.
19. Stoddard Davenport et al., Access Across America: State-by-State Insights into the Accessibility of Care for Mental Health and Substance Use Disorders. Seattle, WA: Milliman, 2023. www.inseparable.us.
20. Quoted in Carla Cantor, "The ER: A Safe Place to Be in a Psychiatric Crisis," Columbia University Department of Psychiatry, September 11, 2023. www.columbiapsychiatry.org.
21. Quoted in Nina Chamlou, "Therapists Who Don't Accept Insurance," Psychology.org, August 15, 2024. www.psychology.org.
22. Joshua Gordon, "Addressing Disparities: Advancing Mental Health Care for All Americans," National Institute of Mental Health, January 29, 2020. www.nimh.nih.gov.
23. American Psychological Association, "Apology to People of Color for APA's Role in Promoting, Perpetuating, and Failing to Challenge Racism, Racial Discrimination, and Human Hierarchy in U.S." October 29, 2021. www.apa.org.

Chapter Three: Mental Illness and Violence

24. Tori DeAngelis, "Mental Illness and Violence: Debunking Myths, Addressing Realities," *Monitor on Psychology*, April 1, 2021. www.apa.org.
25. Chelsea Halle et al., "The Link Between Mental Health, Crime and Violence," *New Ideas in Psychology*, August 2020. www.sciencedirect.com.
26. Tori DeAngelis, "Mental Illness and Violence."

27. Freddie deBoer, "The Case for Forcing the Mentally Ill into Treatment," *New York*, June 20, 2024. nymag.com.
28. Olayemi Olurin, "Jordan Neely Killing: Debates About Mental Health, Crime Are Misguided," *Teen Vogue*, May 12, 2023. www.teenvogue.com.
29. Quoted in Katie O'Connor, "Stigma Linking Mental Illness, Violence Has Increased, Study Finds," *Psychiatric News*, November 6, 2019. https://psychiatryonline.org.
30. Sherry Glied and Richard G. Frank, "Mental Illness and Violence: Lessons from the Evidence," *American Journal of Public Health*, February 2014. https://pmc.ncbi.nlm.nih.gov.
31. Quoted in Matt Shipman, "Study Shows Mentally Ill More Likely to Be Victims, Not Perpetrators, of Violence," NC State University News, February 25, 2014. https://news.ncsu.edu.

Chapter Four: Mental Illness and Homelessness

32. Aaron Lai, "The 'Crushing' Cycle of Homelessness and Mental Illness," Breaktime, May 28, 2021. www.breaktime.org.
33. Quoted in Margaret E. Hampson et al., "Beliefs About Employment of People Living with Psychosis," *Australian Journal of Psychology*, May 2, 2016. www.tandfonline.com.
34. Robert E. Drake and Michael A. Wallach, "Employment Is a Critical Mental Health Intervention," *Epidemiology and Psychiatric Sciences*, November 5, 2020. www.cambridge.org.
35. Quoted in Rick Paulas, "This Is Why Homeless People Don't Go to Shelters," *Vice*, July 24, 2024. www.vice.com.
36. Ashley Womble, "My Homeless Brother's Real Problem Wasn't a Lack of Shelters," *Newsweek*, April 25, 2024. www.newsweek.com.
37. Ayesha Rascoe and Caroline Lewis, "A New Policy in New York City Makes It Easier for Homeless People to Be Forcibly Hospitalized," NPR, December 4, 2022. www.npr.org.
38. April Dembosky et al., "When Homelessness and Mental Illness Overlap, Is Forced Treatment Compassionate?," NPR, March 31, 2023. www.npr.org.

FOR FURTHER RESEARCH

Books

John Allen, *Mental Illness and Homelessness*. San Diego, CA: ReferencePoint, 2025.

Carlin Barnes and Marketa Wills, *Understanding Mental Illness: A Comprehensive Guide to Mental Health Disorders for Family and Friends*. New York: Skyhorse, 2019.

Roy R. Grinker, *Nobody's Normal: How Culture Created the Stigma of Mental Illness*. New York: Norton, 2021.

Mental Health America, *Where to Start: A Survival Guide to Anxiety, Depression, and Other Mental Health Challenges*. New York: Rocky Pond, 2023.

Melanie Siebert and Belle Wuthrich, *Heads Up: Changing Minds on Mental Health*. Victoria, British Columbia, Canada: Orca, 2020.

Internet Sources

Avery Hurt, "How Ancient Societies Viewed Mental Illness and the Horrific Treatments of That Time," *Discover*, September 18, 2024. www.discovermagazine.com.

Audrey Jensen et al., "Two Cities Tried to Fix Homelessness, Only One Succeeded," Cronkite News, December, 14 2020. https://cronkitenews.azpbs.org.

Tana Kelley, "Mental Health May Have Been a Factor in Fatal Shooting of Man's Father, Friend Says," KHQ, February 16, 2022. www.khq.com.

Anna Ross et al., "Media Reporting on Mental Illness, Violence and Crime Needs to Change," The Conversation, August 24, 2020. https://theconversation.com.

Substance Abuse and Mental Health Services Administration, "Mental Health Myths and Facts," April 24, 2023. www.samhsa.gov.

Organizations and Websites

American Psychiatric Association (APA)
www.psychiatry.org

The APA is the world's leading organization of research and treating psychiatrists in the world. Its website offers authoritative information on mental illnesses, along with Psychiatric News, an online journal that shares new developments and research in the field.

KFF
www.kff.org

KFF, formerly the Kaiser Family Foundation, is the United States' leading health policy organization. Its website provides access to poll results tracking health care access and information about the impact of elections and legislation on health care.

Medical News Today
www.medicalnewstoday.com

Medical News Today offers trusted information related to both physical and mental health. It reports on new clinical research, studies, and scientific discoveries in the medical field.

National Alliance on Mental Illness
www.nami.org

This mental health advocacy organization provides vetted information about mental illnesses, treatment options, screening tools, helplines, and other resources. It also coordinates support groups for those suffering from mental illnesses and family groups for friends and family members that meet in locations across the United States.

Psychology Today
www.psychologytoday.com

Psychology Today offers many authoritative articles on a variety of topics related to psychology and mental health. Its noted authors are psychologists and experts in related fields, such as psychiatrists, neuroscientists, and licensed therapists.

INDEX

Note: Boldface page numbers indicate illustrations.

Access Across America, 30
Adams, Eric, 54
Addy, Peter H., 30
adolescent conduct disorder, 35
Affordable Care Act (2010), 28
alcohol abuse disorders and homelessness, 47
American Psychiatric Association, 9, 11, 36
American Psychological Association, 15, 16, 20, 26, 32
Americans with Disabilities Act (1990), 19
anosognosia, 51
antidepressants, 22
antipsychotics, 22
antisocial personality disorder, 35, 36
anxiety disorders
  percentage of Americans with, 12
  percentage of LGBTQ population with, 33
  symptoms of, 12
  treatment for, 23
Australian Journal of Psychiatry, 49
Avery, 5

behavioral health specialists. *See* mental health professionals
Biblical Counseling movement, 11
bipolar disorder
  employment and, 49–50
  medications for, 22
  psychosis as symptom of, 35
brain tumors, 35, **36**
Breaktime, 47–48

"Case for Forcing the Mentally Ill into Treatment, The" (deBoer), 40
catatonia, 35
Centers for Disease Control and Prevention, 12
Charles Schwab modern wealth survey, 47
Chen, Marian, 39
cognitive behavioral therapy (CBT), 16, 23
command hallucinations, 35
confirmation bias, 41–42
COVID-19, 21, 33

deBoer, Freddie, 40
delusions, 35, 51
Denver, Colorado, 43
depression
  homelessness and, 47
  medical treatment for physical problems and, 20
  percentage of Americans experiencing, 11
  percentage of LGBTQ population experiencing, 33
  substance abuse and, 9
  symptoms of, 11–12
  treatment for, 22, 23
Desmarais, Sarah, 43
diagnosis
  disclosure of, 19
  employment and disclosure of, 19
  making, 9–11
  race and, 31–32
  social media and self-, 16–18
Diagnostic and Statistical Manual of Mental Disorders (DSM-5, American Psychiatric Association), 11
discrimination
  in employment, 12, 19
  in health care, 19–20
Dresden (teenager), 17

East Tennessee State University, 38
eating disorders, treatment for, 23
Elbogen, Eric B., 38
employment, **12**
  discrimination in, 12, 19
  homelessness and, 4, 47, 52
  importance of, 49, 50, **50**
  rate of individuals with mental illness compared to those without, 14
  stereotypes, 49–50
  substance abuse disorders and, 19
Epidemiology and Psychiatric Sciences (journal), 50
Erdreich, Sarah, 4–5
eugenics theories, 31, 32

Fonseca, Esperanza, 51–52
Frank, Richard G., 42

Glied, Sherry, 42
Global Burden of Diseases, Injuries, and Risk Factors Study, 48
Gordon, Joshua, 30–31
Gutwinski, Stefan, 46–47

hallucinations, 35, 51
Harrington, Anne, 22
Harris Poll, 20
Health Affairs (journal), 41
health care, discrimination in, 19–20
health insurance, 28–30, 33
Health Resources and Services Administration (HRSA), 25
homeless individuals/homelessness, **48**
  cities' approaches to, 54–55
  criminalization of, 52–53
  employment and, 4, 47, 52

62

Housing First approach, 55
increase in (2019–2023), 47
medications and, 51
Neely murder and, 40
percentage of, with mental illness, 46–47
public opinion about, 53–54
shelters for, 51–52
stigma of, 6
stress and mental illness and, 47–48
teenagers as, 47
treatment and, 30, 31, **32**
hospital emergency rooms, 25, 26–27
Housing First approach to homelessness, 55
Houston, Texas, 55

information and social media, 15–16
inpatient treatment, 23–24
insanity and mental illness, 7

Journal of Medical Internet Research, 16

Karp, Veronica, 20
Katzenstein, Jennifer, 17–18

Lawrence, Ryan, 27
Lawrie, Stephen, 39
Lewis, Caroline, 54
LGBTQ population, 33
Luciano, Alison, 14

MacArthur Violence Risk Assessment Study, 36
Madness in Civilization (Scull), 13
Marano, Hara Estroff, 10
Meara, Ellen, 14
Medicaid, 33
Medical News Today (website), 14
medications, **24**
homelessness and, 51
obtaining, 22, 28
stigma of, 22
types of, 22
mental health
crises response teams, 43, 44

physical health and, 5, 9, 14
Mental Health Parity and Addiction Equity Act (2008), 28
mental health professionals
diagnosis of mental illness by, 9–11
health insurance reimbursement and, 28–29
as members of crisis teams, 43, 44
practitioners of color, 32–33
shortage of, 24–27, **27**
types of
licensed therapists, 9
psychiatrists
abilities of, 9
decrease in number of, 21, 22
religious beliefs and, 11
psychologists, 9, 11, 25
mental illness, **10**
defined, 9
early beliefs about, 13
insanity and, 7
percentage of Americans suffering from, 9
types of, 12–13
See also anxiety disorders; depression
Milliman, 24, 25, 28, 30
mobile medical units, 4
Monitor on Psychology, 35
mood stabilizers, 22

National Epidemiologic Survey on Alcohol and Related Conditions, 37–38
National Health Interview Survey (2023, Centers for Disease Control and Prevention), 12
National Institute of Mental Health, 35
National Stigma Survey, 41
National Survey on Drug Use and Health, 9, 11, 14
Neely, Jordan, **40**, 40–41
New Ideas in Psychology, 37
news media, portrayals of mentally ill as violent, 15, 38–40

confirmation bias and, 41–42
examples of, 34, **40**, 40–41
New York (magazine), 40
New York City, 54
NPR, 55

Olurin, Olayemi, 40–41

paranoia, 35, 51
Penny, Daniel, 40, 41
persecutory delusions, 35
Pescosolido, Bernice, 41
Peteet, John R., 11
Pew Research Center, 15
pharmacotherapy. *See* medications
physical health
depression and medical treatment for, 20
mental health and, 5, 9, 14
police, 43, 44
primary care physicians, 21, 22, 28
psychiatric hospitals, 5
Psychiatric Services (journal), 11
psychiatrists
abilities of, 9
decrease in number of, 21, 22
religious beliefs and, 11
psychologists, 9
religious beliefs and, 11
shortage of, 25
psychotherapy, 22, 30
psychotic disorders
basic facts about, 12, 13, 35
employment and, 49–50
medications for, 22
symptoms of, 35, 51
See also schizophrenia

race, diagnosis and treatment and, 29, 30–32
Reed, James, 4
religious beliefs and treatment, 11, 13, 29
research and race, 31
residential treatment, 23–24

schizoaffective disorder, 35

63

schizophrenia
    employment and, 49–50
    forced hospitalization of those suffering from, 41
    homelessness and, 47
    medications for, 22
    symptoms of, 12–13, 35, 51, 52, 53
Schreiter, Stefanie, 46–47
Scull, Andrew, 13
Semple, Mandy Chapman, 55
shelters for homeless individuals, 51–52
social media, **19**
    information on, 15–16
    self-diagnosis and treatment, 16–18
    as tool to raise awareness and create community, 18
stereotypes
    accessing treatment and, 7
    of Black Americans and professional mental health assistance, 29
    consequences of, 9
    employment and, **12**, 49–50
    examples of, 6–7
    misinformation and, 18
    violence as characteristic of mentally ill, 6, 15
    willpower and recovery, 14
stigma of mental illness
    language used by public officials, 6–7
    of medications for, 22
    relationships and, 20
    treatment and, 17
stress from being homeless, 47–48
substance abuse and depression, 9
Substance Abuse and Mental Health Services Administration, 25, 26
substance abuse disorders, 19, 38
Support Team Assisted Response, 43
Supreme Court, 52–53
Surya, Putri, 8

symptoms
    antisocial personality disorder, 35
    of anxiety disorders, 12
    of bipolar disorder, 35
    of depression, 11–12
    hiding, 19
    of paranoia, 35
    of schizophrenia, 12–13, 35, 51, 52, 53

teenagers
    adolescent conduct disorder, 35
    homeless, 47
    percentage of American, experiencing depressive episodes, 11
    percentage of American, suffering from substance abuse disorders/mental illness, 9
    social media and self-diagnosis by, 16–18
Teen Vogue (magazine), 40–41
TikTok as source of information, 15, 16
treatment, **6**
    barriers to accessing
        costs, 5, 26, 28–30
        lack of sufficient practitioners and facilities, 24–27, **27**
        stereotypes of people with mental illness and, 7
    facilities
        hospital emergency rooms, 25, 26–27
        mentally ill as victims of violence while in, 42–44
        mobile medical units, 4
        psychiatric hospitals, 5
        residential, 23–24
    health insurance coverage for, 20
    homelessness and, 30, 31, **32**
    of LGBTQ population, 33
    race and, 29, 30–31
    religion and, 11, 13, 29
    screening for, 21

    social media and, 16–17
    stigma of mental illness and, 17
    types of
        CBT, 16, 23
        forced hospitalization, 41
        inpatient, 23–24
        medications, 22, **24**, 28, 51
        psychotherapy, 22
        residential, 23–24
Trump, Donald, 41–42
Twitter, as source of information, 15
Tyler, Jeremy, 16

US Census Bureau, 25
US Department of Housing and Urban Development (HUD), 46, 47
US Equal Employment Opportunity Commission, 19

violence
    correlation of mental illness with, 35–38
    crises response teams and, 43
    mentally ill as victims of, **40**, 40–41, 42–44, **44**
    news media portrayals of mentally ill and, 15, 38–40
        confirmation bias and, 41–42
        examples of, 34, **40**, 40–41
        in shelters for homeless individuals, 52
        statements by authority figures on mentally ill and, 6
    substance abuse disorders and, 38

Washington Post, 44
Womble, Ashley, 52
World Psychiatry (journal), 22

Yale University, 38
Yeiser, Bethany, 53